# Intermittent Fasting:

*Step-by-Step Guide to Lose Weight Rapidly and Eat Healthy with Keto Diet — Heal Your Body with Autophagy. Use the Best Mindset for Succeed in Fasting Easily for Wellness and Longevity*

by ALAN DIETER

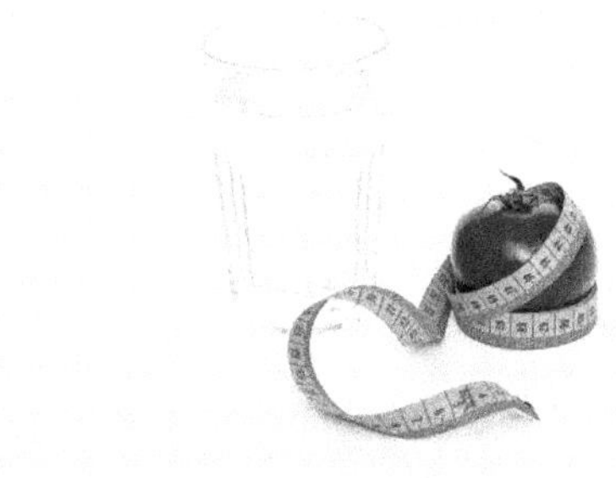

# Table of Contents

# Introduction

Congratulations on purchasing *Intermittent Fasting*, and thank you for doing so!

Are you looking for the most effective way to lose weight and maintain optimal health? Intermittent fasting is the answer to your search. This book is a great resource if you are interested in combining intermittent fasting and keto but are unsure about where to begin.

Inside this book, you will find invaluable information on how you can use intermittent fasting and the ketogenic diet to bring a turnaround in your life and lose weight as you've never done before.

This book focuses on how you can combine the ketogenic diet and intermittent fasting for the best results. It first begins by looking at intermittent fasting in-depth, followed up by all the basics of the ketogenic diet. We take a look at the different intermittent fasting methods, as well as how to fit the ketogenic diet into intermittent fasting.

Intermittent fasting takes a closer look at both intermittent fasting and the ketogenic diet to give you an exciting solution to weight loss. This looks at the different aspects of both intermittent fasting and the ketogenic diet to help you understand the mechanism of these two diets before you can even think of combining them.

The book particularly looks at the workings of each diet; hence, it will help you to make the decision to lead a life full of vitality. Whether you are interested in losing weight or you simply desire to lead a healthy lifestyle, this book offers you detailed information, complete with how to make a smooth transition so that you're able to adhere to the plan.

Combining a low-carb diet with intermittent fasting will certainly usher you into a new health perspective. By the time you finish reading this book, you will be sufficiently equipped with all the information you need to begin combining intermittent fasting and the ketogenic diet and enjoy all the benefits that it offers. I believe this book will mark the beginning of a new chapter in your lifestyle.

# Chapter 1:

# What Is Intermittent Fasting?

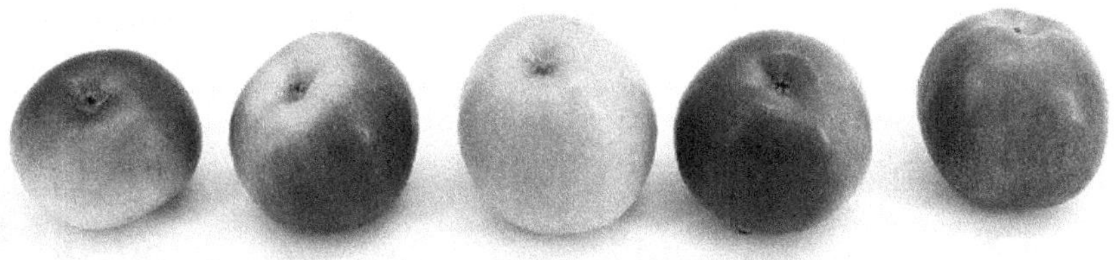

When you talk about fasting, what comes to mind for most people is starvation. This is a huge misconception because intermittent fasting is actually a lifestyle. It involves going without food deliberately and voluntarily, for a specified duration, and alternating it with a specific window of time within which you can eat. You can practice intermittent fasting for various reasons, although most people who embrace it are motivated by the numerous benefits that result from calorie restriction.

What sets intermittent fasting from other forms of fasting like religious fasting or a diagnostic fast is the fact that you are at liberty to take fluids and non-caloric beverages during the fasting window. This makes fasting bearable and easy to follow through while still reaping the benefits.

## History of Fasting

Fasting is an age-old practice that has been in existence since the time of the agrarian revolution. At the time, human beings who were mostly hunters and gatherers were forced to fast owing to the scarcity of food. Without cold storage or even modern food preservation technology, they would eat whenever they found adequate food and go without food for long periods in times of scarcity. Yet, others fasted for medical and religious reasons.

Hippocrates, a Greek philosopher and the father of modern medicine, also advocated for fasting for medical reasons. According to Hippocrates, eating while you are sick is equivalent to feeding the sickness because disease-causing microorganisms are able to thrive. He argued that animals didn't eat while they were sick, and this contributed to their speedy healing besides improving their cognitive function. Plutarch and Plato equally advocated for this. Greeks believed that this same principle could apply to human beings. This concept has been integrated into modern medicine; thus, it's a common practice to find patients who are due for surgery being put on compulsory fast hours before the procedure.

Fasting has also been practiced as a spiritual practice in different religions. For instance, Muslims do practice Ramadhan in fulfillment of the fifth pillar of Islam. They take time to pray and reflect. Christians, too, set aside time to pray and fast as a way of seeking spiritual benefits.

## History of Intermittent Fasting

Intermittent fasting is not an entirely new concept from ancient fasting patterns. The only new thing about intermittent fasting is the clinical research linking this practice to numerous health benefits and longevity that is driving many people to embrace it. In fact, one of the reasons why intermittent fasting continues to gain popularity is because it's one of the few diets that actually produces results and has the backing of scientific evidence. Intermittent fasting was first popularized in 2012 by BBC journalist and doctor Michael Mosley after sharing the outcome of his two-week journey of the 5:2 protocol. Dr. Mosley shared the benefits of the fasting protocol on his TV program that included rapid weight loss. He went on two write a book, hence making intermittent fasting popular.

To date, millions of people have embraced this practice that continues to produce results. This is partly because of the flexibility of this practice as you get to choose a fasting protocol that is suitable for your lifestyle and needs. Moreover, intermittent fasting is easy to follow since you're simply adjusting your feeding hours, which your body gets accustomed to through time, thus making it doable.

## Who Can Practice Intermittent Fasting?

Intermittent fasting is not exclusive to health enthusiasts because we all practice this pattern of eating in one way or the other. Think about the hours you are awake and the number of hours you spend sleeping. These intervals can rightly fit into the fasting and feasting windows keeping in mind the time you have your first and last meal. The only distinguishing factor is the fact that when you practice intermittent fasting, you're more deliberate about the length of your fast.

Generally, nearly everyone can practice intermittent fasting apart from people who have special needs. However, you must make sure that your intermittent fasting plan is well structured if you're to achieve the results you desire. Most importantly, you must be ready to adhere to your intermittent fasting plan. You can practice intermittent fasting if; you are single with no children, you have been watching your food and calorie consumption, you have a good support system, and your job allows you periods of low performance. Although you can also follow intermittent fasting if you are in complete sports, have a performance-oriented job are married with children, you must do so with caution.

# Who Shouldn't Practice Intermittent Fasting

Although intermittent fasting is simply a pattern of

eating, not everyone can practice it because it can result in some inconveniences or introduce risks that outweigh the benefits for some people. You shouldn't practice intermittent fasting if:

- *You're below 18 years.* The reason for this is simple. At 18 years, you're growing actively; hence, your body requires all the minerals and vital vitamins that promote growth and development. Therefore, intermittent fasting will be counterproductive.

- *You're expectant or nursing.* Nursing and expectant mothers should not practice intermittent fasting because their bodies are providing nourishment for the baby. Besides, your body needs more calories when breastfeeding and during pregnancy.

- *You have gastroesophageal reflux disease (GERD).* Various studies have concluded that intermittent fasting can worsen GERD because when you fast, your stomach will be without food for a couple of hours. Therefore, the gastric juices will not have anything to digest except your stomach lining.

- *You're underweight and malnourished.* It's unrealistic to get into intermittent fasting when you're already underweight or are battling an eating disorder because this can only make a bad situation worse.

- *You suffer from chronic stress or have had a history of disordered eating.* You shouldn't practice intermittent fasting, as this comes with a diet pattern of exercise and diet regiment—that means you will not sleep well.

## A Word of Caution

Although intermittent fasting is a pattern of fasting that can be adopted by just about everyone because it's safe, you must approach it with caution for the following reasons:

Not everybody can practice intermittent fasting because of the effect this pattern of eating can have on your physiological functions. Therefore, make sure you talk to a doctor before you begin. This is important because it'll help you to take care of any prevailing health conditions that you may not have been aware existed. Remember, you should not undergo fasting when you're not in good health.

While women are discouraged from practicing intermittent fasting, the reality is that there are certain groups of women who can undergo fasting and reap the benefits of fasting just like their male counterparts. However, you'll need to talk to a doctor, particularly if you're suffering from diabetes, low blood pressure, you're trying to conceive, or have an eating disorder. All these are considered to be risk factors.

## What Happens During Fasting?

When you're following the normal eating pattern, your body depends on glucose from the food that you consume. The rest is stored as fat. When you fast, the body goes into a state known as ketosis, where the liver will break down the fat into ketones that are then used as a source of energy. Evidence suggests that ketones are capable of suppressing appetite while also reducing oxidative stress and inflammation levels. However, keep in mind that ketones offer many other benefits other than the production of energy. Fasting reduces risk factors for conditions such as type 2 diabetes and heart diseases.

## Why Should You Practice Intermittent Fasting for Fat Loss?

One of the things that have drawn so many people to intermittent fasting is the fact that you can achieve weight loss with this pattern of eating. If you've already practiced numerous diet fads without any results, intermittent fasting could just be the solution you've been looking for as long as you practice it as required. So why should you practice intermittent fasting for fat loss? First, you need to know that intermittent fasting is not a tangible product but a process that involves a lifestyle change, especially with regard to your relationship with food. It's a natural process that lets your body burn fat and lose weight through calorie restriction. However, unlike other diets that require you to count your calories, this diet restricts calories by reducing the duration within which you're allowed to it. So, you will naturally consume fewer calories than you would when following a normal eating pattern. When this happens, you experience a calorie deficit that means that your body must then tap into the fat stores to be able to make up for the deficit. The result of this is the loss of fat because the stored fat is broken down to produce energy for the body.

Secondly, intermittent fasting has continued to gain traction as more and more people across the world share their experiences and results of following this eating pattern. The reason is simple. Unlike many diets that are expensive and difficult to follow through, intermittent fasting is simple, easy to follow, yet it produces results. Anyone can start and follow through intermittent fasting without necessarily having to change your diet. This eating pattern is also not restrictive rather so that you go back to your old eating habits at the end of the diet; rather, it's more of a change in lifestyle, so it's something you can adopt in the long term.

Lastly, intermittent fasting is easy to follow and more relaxed because the only restriction is the window during which you fast and feast. That is, it emphasizes on the number of hours when you need to eat and when you need to fast. However, you'll be allowed to take water and beverages as long as they are calorie-free. This helps in suppressing the urge to eat or crave certain foods.

Moreover, you'll be able to burn more fat so that you become healthier and leaner. Intermittent fasting is a holistic way of leading a healthy lifestyle.

## Why Should You Start Intermittent Fasting?

If you have heard about intermittent fasting for some time now, you must be wondering whether you should join the bandwagon or not. Well, unless you have a prevailing medical condition, you can be sure to follow intermittent fasting successfully. Your body is well conditioned to handle long periods without food. In fact, you'll be surprised that you can go up to 84 hours without food before you can begin to experience a significant drop in your glucose levels. So many changes occur in the body during fasting, most of which have a positive influence on your overall wellness.

Fasting does pave the way for a number of repair processes that target the genes, hormones, and cells. During fasting, your body's insulin levels decrease significantly while the human growth hormone increases. Intermittent fasting also increases your metabolic health benefits because it improves the number of risk factors and health markers. When you fast, your lifespan also increases because fasting has been found to increase longevity, especially through a process known as autophagy. You can also practice intermittent fasting for the simple reason that it makes your day simple since you no longer have to spend hours preparing meals and eating. While you'd have to prepare up to six meals on any given day, intermittent fasting reduces this time because, in some instances, you may just need to prepare two meals. Most important of all is that the human body has the capacity to adapt to such changes. After all, it echoes the way of life of an early man who ate when there was plenty and fasted during the times of scarcity. There are many reasons why you should start practicing intermittent today. You'll be surprised at the tremendous changes that you'll experience apart from weight and fat loss that are easily noticeable.

# Chapter 2:

# Common Intermittent Fasting Methods

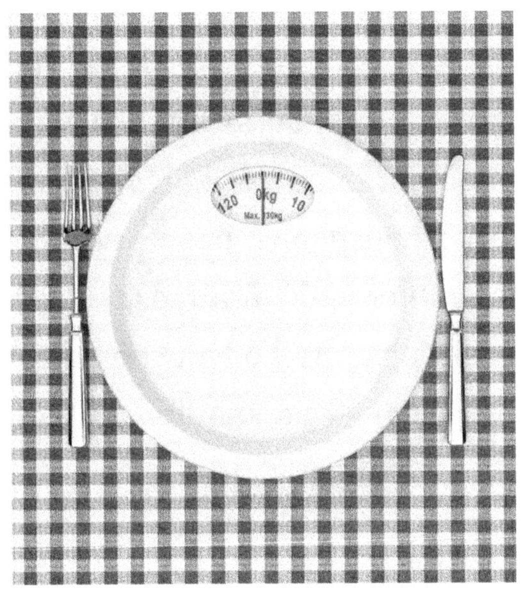

There are numerous ways to do intermittent fasting. These methods vary in terms of the calorie allowances and the number of days/hours that you can do them. Depending on the method that you choose, intermittent fasting may involve fasting partially so that you only eat for a set amount of time or fasting entirely for a whole day before you can resume eating regularly. Since every person has a different experience with intermittent fasting, different styles will appeal to different people. In this chapter, we discuss the common intermittent fasting methods of doing intermittent fasting.

## The 16:8 Method – The Leangains Method

With this method of intermittent fasting, you'll be required to fast for 16 hours and only have an eating window of 8 hours, hence 16:8. It's the most common fasting protocol because most people are already used to going without food for long durations, especially at night. A Swedish nutritionist and bodybuilder, Martin Berkhan, created this method. This method is easy to adopt, especially if you're already used to a 12-hour fasting period. However, women can do a modification of this method by fasting for 14 hours with a 10-hour feeding window. When followed properly, this method maximizes your muscle while cutting on fat. This method is complemented by a light workout that is mainly strength training. What is even interesting is that the creator of this intermittent fasting method does not only focus on weight loss but also muscle building and body re-composition. The 16:8 Method is not a one-size-fits-all; thus, you're free to adapt it to your needs, especially with regard to meal timing and macro-nutrient breakdown. It's easy to make this method your lifestyle over time.

## Following the 16:8 Method

For you to be successful with the 16:8 intermittent fasting method, you must be ready to keep a journal to track your progress. This can be a challenge if journaling is not something you do regularly. Yet this is important in helping you to not only track but also achieve the results you desire. You're free to determine when you will eat and when you will fast. Berkhan suggests that you begin your feasting window in the afternoon all the way to half-past eight because this will ensure that you don't miss out on social gathering where you have to eat. After all, this is when the social scene is active, and it is followed by the first hours of your fast that you will spend while sleeping that you're already accustomed to. The interesting about this method is that you'll have to skip breakfast that has been argued to be the most important meal of the day. Additionally, you have to set aside a time when you will do your workout to which Berkhan suggests the following options; you can opt to do your workout as soon as you wake up or work out after your first meal into the feasting window. You could also opt to work out after your second meal. You should make sure that you target your workouts to focus on strength training while limiting your meal times to three during the 8-hour feasting window. The reason for this is simple. It's not easy to have more than three meals in just about 8 hours. However, make sure you have a large post-workout meal with over sixty percent of your recommended daily calorie intake coming from this meal. The reason behind this is simple; your body is accustomed to converting food into muscle post-workout. Therefore, refrain from practicing fasted training because it's taxing and puts you at risk of suffering from bur out. When this happens, you could end up needing to take supplements, which means you have more things to track. As such, it's better to maintain working out during your feasting window. This also helps you to have quality sleep since your body will be physically tired. Ultimately, make sure you maintain a calorie deficit or just eat at maintenance.

For you to know the number of calories you need, begin

by calculating your Basal Metabolic Rate (BMR) so that you're sure about the number of calories you need to maintain your current weight. Make sure you consider your activity level when calculating your BMR. Unless you're sedentary, make sure you pick the level where you're at or go a level lower. Desist from the common mistake of underestimating your activity level because a deficit means five hundred calories less this number, and the maintenance is a similar number of calories. Therefore, when you eat the specified number of calories, you'll be able to maintain your current weight. When you carefully follow the 16:8 fasting method along with the workout, your body will undergo immense re-composition, replacing fat with muscle. Don't be discouraged if you have to lose so much weight in order to reach your healthy weight. You'll definitely begin to see the results over time when you start losing fat, and your muscle becomes dense.

It's also important to think about the food you will be eating as well as the proportions. To do this, take advantage of the online calculators to estimate the size of your food portions and calories you need so you know how to distribute them across the three meals. You also need to determine the proportion of your food that will be carbohydrates and what proportion will comprise proteins. Should you opt to incorporate the ketogenic diet, make sure that you include a higher proportion of fat compared to carbs. You don't have to worry about putting on weight from consuming fats because your insulin levels decrease during fasting, thereby promoting the burning of fat. Carbs are important, especially during your workout, because they help in fueling your muscles. If you realize that you're following through this plan, but you're still not able to realize any significant weight loss, you will have to reduce your daily caloric intake by at least 500 calories and continue journaling the progress.

## Making Your 16:8 Intermittent Fasting Method a Success

Although this intermittent fasting protocol is popular, it's not easy to follow through. However, you can follow these tips to be able to post excellent results:

- This program requires that you work out with the emphasis being strength training.

- Make sure you include a sufficient proportion of proteins in the meals you consume during the fasting period.

- Make sure your meals are nutrient-dense while staying away from calorie bombs that add little or no nutritional value.

- Don't consume any calories within the feasting window. This includes anything with the potential of causing your insulin levels to spike. Instead, focus on drinking lots of water and other non-caloric beverages to stay hydrated.

- Avoid eating pre-workout, but instead, have a large post-workout meal.

In conclusion, while intermittent fasting is not about calorie restriction, taking fewer carbs will make the 16:8 Method a huge success.

## Pros of the 16:8 Method

- This intermittent fasting pattern tends to offer structure to your day owing to the consistency of the fasting/feasting window.

- This method is planned with physical activity in mind, so it will work well if you lead an active lifestyle.

- The fasting window of this method is not so extreme, like a majority of other fasting diets, making it so easy to stick to.

## Cons of the 16:8 Method

- Some people may not want to cycle their carb and calorie intake.

- For optimal results, Berkhan recommends that you need to train when you're in the fasted state. This is impractical for those people who prefer to train later. Even then, you can find different templates on how you can apply this method in various scenarios.

## The 5:2 Method – Eat Stop Eat

Eat Stop Eat is the intermittent fasting method that propelled the intermittent fasting method into popularity after Dr. Mosley shared the results of his two-week fast.

However, this pattern of eating is originally the brainchild of Brad Pilon, a bodybuilder. This plan is designed to imitate the ancient lifestyle that was practiced by the hunting and gathering communities. Interestingly, you will not find a lot of information on this intermittent fasting plan online. This is in no way meant to mean that this method is not effective because you'll be amazed by the kind of results you'll post with this method of fasting.

Are you wondering what this intermittent fasting method entails? Well, with the eat stop eat method, you get to eat regularly for 5 days and set aside two days of fasting. This means you'll have two 24-hour blocks during which you shouldn't consume any calories. This can be a little difficult for most people, but it can be done because you can still take fluids that do not contain calories. The major misgiving with this intermittent fasting method is that you could end up binge eating after going for 24 hours without food. Even then, studies have discredited this, arguing that the excess calories you'll consume after your fast don't qualify to make it binge eating. All in all, you'll do well to distribute the days you'll be fasting realistically to have a realistic gap so that you don't end up binge eating at the end of the fast.

# How to Do the 5:2 Intermittent Fasting Method

Although fasting for 24 hours is not for the faint-hearted, the 5:2 Method can be a good place to start the intermittent fasting lifestyle. The reason is simple; the rules governing this method of fasting are not too harsh. In addition, this method also has minimal requirements, so it's easy for anyone to start on it, including beginners. Although Brad Pilon recommends complimenting this method with exercises, it doesn't have to be HIIT or strength training as long as you're able to break a move and sweat.

You'll do well to know where you stand in terms of maintenance calories, even though this is not a must because you can balance this out on the days when you're not fasting. This is good motivation because beginners can be encouraged to carry on without being under too much pressure yet attain the desired weight loss. However, you need to realize that the weight loss associated with this method is not as rapid as with other intermittent fasting methods. Moreover, you have to follow the guidelines keenly to achieve results.

Unfortunately, beginners are often the greatest victims of flouting the guidelines because of lacking a good understanding of the nutritional component resulting in discouragement and eventually abandoning the program. This is also a major shortcoming of this program.

## Sample 5:2 Setup

- Monday – Normal eating

- Tuesday – Up to 500 / 600 calories

- Wednesday – Normal eating

- Thursday – Normal eating

- Friday – 500 / 600 calories

- Saturday – Normal eating

- Sunday – Normal eating

## The Pros of 5:2

- This method of fasting can suit certain categories of people psychologically.

- You don't have to track your calorie consumption.

# The Cons of 5:2

- This method of fasting may not be suitable for people who are in jobs that require them to be active.

- It can be difficult to stick to this plan in the long term.

- Since you have no restrictions on calorie consumption, you can easily overeat on the days when you eat normally.

# The Warrior Method

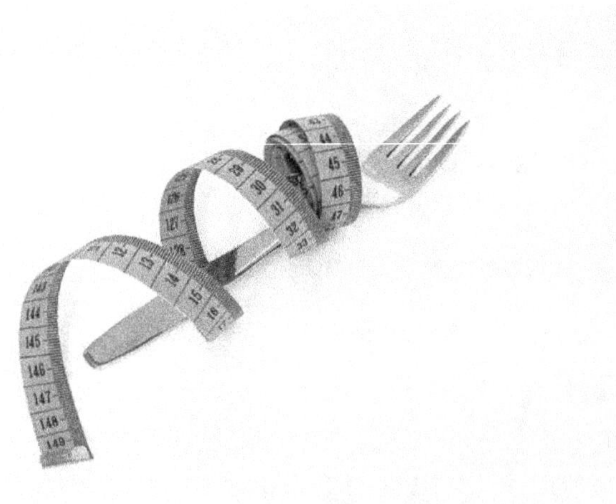

The warrior method of intermittent fasting is relatively

extreme of all the intermittent fasting methods because you have to fast for 20 hours and eat for 4 hours. As such, it is recommended for those who have already experimented with the other intermittent fasting methods. Ori Hofmekler, a former member of the Israeli Special Forces who later transitioned into nutrition and fitness, originally created this method. Following this method to the later will change your perspective on the amount of food you need to eat as well as the frequency of meals that you need for the proper functioning of your body. This method is a lot stricter when compared to the Leangains method because it lengthens the fasting window by four hours while shortening the feeding window by 4 hours. As such, it's likely that you will only be able to have one large meal during the feeding window. Although this doesn't seem practical, this diet will get you the results you so much desire.

The only challenge is that you must make sure you stick to this plan to get the results. This is something most people struggle with. However, it's not difficult to get started on this diet as you can find tons of motivation from the online community of people who have either tried it or are doing it now. It is believed to be practiced by those people with a tough personality. Thus, don't be surprised if you don't get any sympathy or even support if you're struggling with adherence. Overall, your success with this plan is mostly psychological and hence has the potential to have a negative effect on your relationship with food.

## How to Do the Warrior Diet

Before you can even think about beginning your fast under the warrior diet, you must calculate your BMR so you know the number of calories you should get from fat, proteins, and carbs. You need to determine the amount of protein you need, followed by carbs and fats. You also need to come up with a plan on how you'll be working out, keeping in mind your short feasting window. Although you need to work out during the feeding window, this can be a challenge logistically because the amount of time you need for your work out is just about half of your feeding window. Besides, since you have a large meal portion, you need sufficient time to eat to allow digestion to take place. On the other hand, when you work out during your fasting window, you're unlikely to attain optimum performance that will meet the demand for strength training even if you take supplements. The idea here is that after 24 hours of fasting, your body needs proper nutrition. Therefore, attempting to work out while in the fasted state will increase this need. On the other hand, when you work out after a single meal means you'll have inadequate time to eat. Therefore, you need to balance this by shortening the length of your workout to preserve your muscle mass.

In this case, High-Intensity Interval Training (HIIT) is the most ideal as it can push your heart rate up to 90% of its maximum ability within a short time so that you have a slightly longer duration of rest. You can repeat this within 15- to 20-minute intervals. You can engage in any activity as long as you're doing it with great intensity. This can be anything from sprinting to cycling, pushups, squats and jump rope, and so much more. You just need to make sure that you avoid injuries. You can gradually reduce your resting interval as you get used to this plan. However, you must keep in mind that you can only develop strength up to a certain level. In addition, you can't build muscle beyond a certain point.

# Pros of the Warrior Method

- This method will work well for those people who are not hungry during the day, owing to their work schedule, so you find it easier to skip breakfast and eat later in the day.

- Cutting down on your consumption of meals to 1 or 2 meals in a day will help when calories are low.

- This plan mainly emphasizes on eating nutrient-rich, whole foods like vegetables and fruits.

# Cons of the Warrior Method

- The set-up of this method of fasting makes it most likely to have to train in the fasted state that might not be practical.

- This method might not be sustainable for most people.

# Alternate-Day Fasting – 36/12 Fast

Nutritionist and Dr. James B. Johnson designed the alternate-day fasting method. This intermittent fasting method involves fasting every other day and comes in several variations. This method recommends fasting for 36 hours and feeding for 12 hours, but you can do it. Thus, you can have your three meals during the feeding period. While some people will limit their calorie intake to 500 others, practice complete avoidance of food. Since this method of fasting promotes fasting for an extended duration, it's not suitable for beginners. When following this plan, you must have a higher intake of proteins and fats compared to carbs. This method is silent about working out, probably because of the long fasting period. This method is not as strict because it gives you the freedom to eat anything as long as it's a healthy choice. You'll do well to stick to nutrient-dense foods while avoiding calorie-dense foods.

## How to Do the 36/12 Method

Before you start implementing the alternate-day fasting method, you need to begin by defining your feasting and fasting windows. That is establishing when your fasting period will begin and when your feeding window you start. For instance, if your first meal is at 8 am and your last meal at 8 pm on Sunday, you can repeat this schedule at least 4 times each week. Your fasting window typically begins after your last meal of the day.

Many people have posted positive results with alternate-day fasting because it not only promotes weight loss but also contributes to overall well-being. Most people who have strictly followed this plan have recorded weight loss of up to 8 percent within 8 weeks. Other benefits you'll experience with this method of fasting include improved insulin resistance and better cellular energy production. This method is excellent if you want to tap into the benefits of autophagy.

Nonetheless, fasting for 36 hours can be too harsh for the female body; hence, it's recommended that women who want to follow this method have at least 500 calories during the fasting window. You can consider taking smoothies are fruits as these have low calories. Combine this with exercise like strength training to enhance fat burning and obtain better results.

## Alternate-Day Fasting Setup

- Monday – Normal eating

- Tuesday – Up to 500 / 600 calories

- Wednesday – Normal eating

- Thursday – Normal eating

- Friday – 500 / 600 calories

- Saturday – Normal eating

- Sunday – Normal eating

# Pros of Alternate-Day Fasting

Some of the advantages of alternate-day fasting include the following:

- This method of fasting is handy in improving conditions such as asthma.

- Alternate-day fasting extends your lifespan as well as improving metabolism.

- You'll not experience deprivation because you are allowed to eat anything during the feeding window.

- This method is easy to follow in the long term.

- It's good for your health.

- It doesn't have stringent rules as long as you eat healthy meals.

## Cons of Alternate-Day Fasting

The disadvantages of intermittent fasting include:

- You're likely to experience some unpleasant side effects with this method, such as fatigue, dizziness, and hunger, particularly in the beginning.

- This pattern of eating is not good for those people who have a history of eating disorders such as anorexia.

- This method doesn't say anything about exercising or even the role of working out.

## The 12/12 Method

This intermittent fasting pattern is easy to follow because you have an equal length of fasting and feeding duration. That means you're fasting for 12 hours and feeding for another 12 hours. This is quite manageable, keeping in mind that some of those hours of your fasting window will be spent sleeping. Therefore, you hardly get to feel hungry. The only challenge is that you need to limit your meal times to a maximum of three within the 12 hours of feeding. So you can opt for an equal feeding interval, so you don't have to eat snacks in between meals. A 12-hour fast is great because it allows your system sufficient time to rest. Besides, it contributes to a decline in your insulin levels, thus promoting weight loss. Nonetheless, you shouldn't be surprised if you still experience uneasiness, nausea, or a slight headache in the initial stages of fasting because it will take time before your body can adjust. This reaction is usually a result of the withdrawal of sugar, so your body tries to adjust to this change. Like the other intermittent fasting protocols, you need to stay hydrated by taking lots of water and drinks that don't have calories.

## Crescendo Fasting

The crescendo method of intermittent fasting was designed for women because of the female body's sensitivity to signals of starvation. For most women, fasting triggers hormonal imbalances that are translated as hunger pangs. Fatigue, mood swings, and weight gain. The crescendo method of fasting is less demanding, making it suitable. When you practice this method of fasting, you don't have to fast daily rather you fast for 12-16 hours per day for up to 3 non-consecutive days weekly. This means that you're still able to maintain your regular feeding plan on those days when you're not fasting. You also must refrain from heavy workouts but consider yoga and cardio. Intense exercises like strength training and HIIT are also recommended.

## Pros of Crescendo Fasting

- This method is great when you want to burn fat pockets and slim without having to embrace a demanding routine.

- This method is gentle on the female body; thus, it helps in preserving the hormonal balance that is important for a woman's body.

- Crescendo fasting is an excellent way of preparing your body to handle the complicated intermittent fasting methods like the warrior method and eat stop eat among others.

# Cons of Crescendo Fasting

- This method of fasting is not recommended for people with eating disorders because it'll make it worse.

- Practicing this method of fasting could result in an irregular menstrual cycle. In the event that this happens, stop fasting immediately.

# Chapter 3:

# How to Do Intermittent Fasting in a Healthy and Safe Way

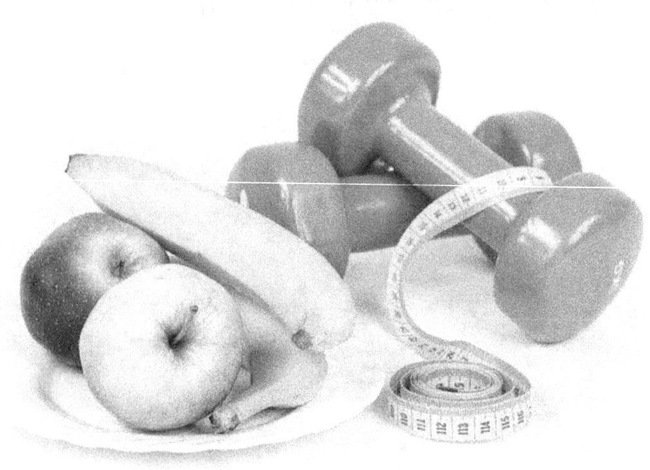

Intermittent fasting is a health trend that is unstoppable because of the evolutionary rationale that drives it. The pattern of eating has been the basis of numerous studies and trials that have sought to investigate the relationship between fasting and its benefits. However, to achieve the benefits, you must practice fasting along with other supporting pillars that include heavy plant nutrition, exercise, mindfulness, and sleep.

One of the concerns of intermittent fasting is how to practice it safely and get to harness all the amazing benefits keeping in mind that you'll be going for long hours without food. A number of intermittent fasting studies done on women have posted overwhelming outcomes of this lifestyle intervention. This is especially true if you're overweight or have a mild metabolic dysfunction like prediabetes and even inflammation. Like any other good thing, too much intermittent fasting can become bad, hence the need to make sure you do it right.

When you talk about doing intermittent fasting in a healthy and safe way, you need to keep in mind that precision is everything. This applies to any other lifestyle intervention as they are all created to be equal and produce a dose-dependent response. When done moderately, intermittent fasting will promote sustainable weight loss, improved lipid levels, reduce inflammation, and improve lipid levels. You'll need to approach intermittent fasting with caution if you are used to engaging in high levels of physical activity. To make sure you're practicing intermittent fasting safely, you need to consider the following:

- *Talk to your doctor or nutritionist.* Anyone can practice intermittent fasting, including people who are living with diabetes. However, you need to make sure you're under the supervision of a medical professional or nutritionist. When you talk to your doctor, you are able to discuss with them the limits so that you know the level you can get to as well as what is off-limits for you. They will also advise you on the fasting method that is best suited for you.

- *Choose a suitable intermittent fasting method.* Once you have been given the green light to proceed with fasting, you need to identify the intermittent fasting method that will work best for you because not all methods are suitable for everyone. One of the things that you need to consider while choosing an intermittent fasting plan is your lifestyle. This includes your work. Choose a plan that compliments your work schedule as well as your goals. While at it, don't be too ambitious as to go for a plan that you can't keep up with because this will only result in you struggling before quitting.

- *Focus on healthy food choices.* Although intermittent fasting doesn't emphasize on the kind of foods you need to eat during the duration you'll be fasting, it's advisable to stick to healthy food choices, especially nutrient-dense foods. These will often leave you feeling full for longer, making it easier to cope with the long hours of fasting. This also makes it possible for you to lose weight if this is your ultimate goal because you will not be feeding on empty calories.

- *Start with the moderate intermittent fasting methods gradually advancing to the more complex plans.* The good thing about intermittent fasting methods is that they have been designed to accommodate the needs of just about every category of people. As a beginner, you will do well by beginning with the friendlier methods of fasting that require you to fast for fewer hours and advance to the more complex methods where you'll be fasting for longer hours.

- *Work out in moderation.* Most of the intermittent fasting methods require you to compliment the fast with workouts. This doesn't mean that you can work out as you would when you are following the normal eating plan. Instead, you should focus your workouts, such that they will coincide with your feeding window, and you can do then in moderation.

- *Keep a positive mindset.* A positive mindset is an important component when you talk about safety in intermittent fasting. When you have the right mentality, you will refrain from the temptation to fast without thinking about your needs.

## Can Intermittent Fasting Be Dangerous?

Despite all the evidence put forth in support of intermittent fasting, you must keep in mind that not all types of intermittent fasting are safe or even supported by scientific evidence. Therefore, even for the intermittent fasting methods that have been tested, you must avoid prolonged fasting for an extended duration, especially beyond 36 hours unless you're doing it for medical reasons and have consulted your physician. Some of the intermittent fasting methods have been popularized by people outside the medical and scientific fields, which is dangerous. This includes dry fasting that doesn't have any scientific backing. There are no human studies that have been done to advance dry fasting, and this form of fasting doesn't promote autophagy, either, and hence must be discouraged. If you must practice any form of fasting, you must make sure that it is backed with scientific evidence or clinical trials that prove it to be safe.

## Safety Concerns About Intermittent Fasting

The main safety concern when doing intermittent fasting is the possibility of malnutrition or undernutrition. Individuals who are underweight and have a nutritional deficiency or are at risk of such need not to practice intermittent fasting. In fact, they shouldn't practice a fast that lasts more than 12 hours. Women may sometimes experience irregular periods or even have issues with their reproductive health. This is often caused by substantive weight loss, accompanied by excessive exercise. Women who are expecting must also not practice intermittent fasting because their nutritional needs are even more during this time. Ultimately, you need to understand that an intermittent fasting schedule that works for one person may not work for another person. Thus, you will do well to evaluate how you fair with the fasts while paying attention to your overall well-being. Some of the things you can do to practice intermittent fasting safely are:

- Make sure you're well-hydrated and drink up whenever you feel thirsty.

- Adjust your calorie consumption during the feasting window to pack up enough calories to meet your weight loss/maintenance goals.

- Go for fasting schedules that let you eat in the light-dark cycle as within your normal circadian rhythm.

- Don't hesitate to break your fast early whenever you feel nauseous, faint, or dizzy.

# Chapter 4:

# Benefits of Intermittent Fasting

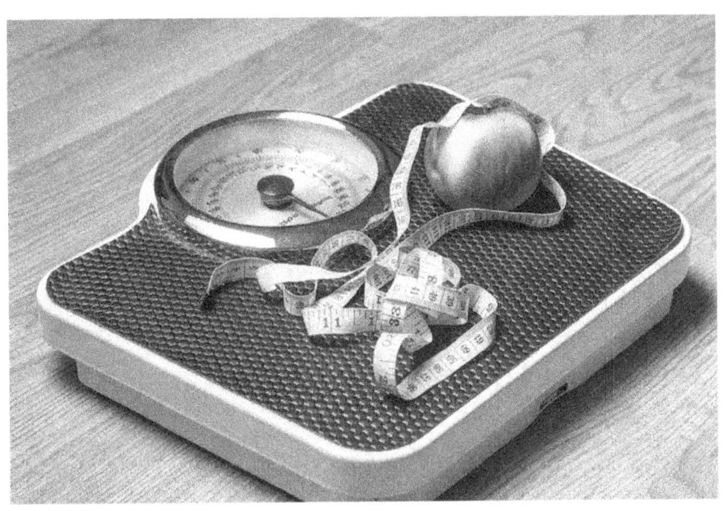

One of the reasons why intermittent fasting continues to gain popularity is because of the many benefits it offers. Moreover, unlike many diets that promise rapid weight loss but only end up to be fads, you can be sure to experience weight loss with intermittent fasting when you do it properly. Some of the benefits of intermittent fasting include the following:

## Intermittent Fasting Prompts Multiple Cellular Processes

Your body is made up of trillions of cells. The cells keep you alive and healthy through a regeneration process. When you fast, your body undergoes a number of physiological processes, including initiation of a cellular regeneration process that is known as autophagy. This process involves metabolization of the broken and dysfunctional proteins that build up within cells over time.

## Intermittent Fasting Does Change the Function of Hormones, Genes, and Cells

When your body is deprived of food for an extended duration, a number of processes are initiated. These changes include cellular repair processes as well as changes in your hormonal levels ostensibly to make the stored fat accessible for conversion into energy. Other important changes that occur are a significant decline in your levels of insulin that also promotes the burning of fat. Your body also experiences an increase in the levels of your growth hormones that also promote fat burning as well as muscle gain. Other cellular repair processes that take place include removing waste material from the cells. You could also experience other beneficial changes that take place in molecules and genes relating to longevity as well as protection against diseases.

## Intermittent Fasting Leads to a Reduction of Inflammation and Oxidative Stress

Oxidative stress is usually pre precursor to aging as well as most chronic diseases. It involves a number of molecules that are known as free radicals. The free radicals react with other useful molecules causing damage to them. Various studies indicate that intermittent fasting will enhance the body's ability to resist oxidative stress. In addition, it will also help in fighting inflammation that is another major driver of diseases.

## Intermittent Fasting Is Therapeutic

The benefits of intermittent fasting go beyond the physical to also offer psychological and spiritual benefits. The physical benefits that you will experience that include a reduction in seizures, an improvement in the symptoms of diabetes, or even a cure for diabetes are well aligned to the spiritual benefits cutting across religions that practice fasting across the globe. When it comes to the psychological benefits, the nature of intermittent fasting prompts you to exercise control of your will power and mind by saying not to food during the fasting window even when you're hungry. This produces a great psychological effect. The ability to exercise restraint and ignore hunger when you're hungry is quite powerful.

## Intermittent Fasting Supports the Production of the Neuron Growth Hormone

When you go for a couple of hours without food, your body begins to operate on a cycle that ketone-based. As such, there will be an increase in the production of the Brain-Derived Neurotropic Factor (BDNF). This refers to a type of protein that is responsible for promoting neuron growth in the brain. This protein also ensures the protection of the neurons from other kinds of damage.

# Intermittent Fasting Enhances Body Building

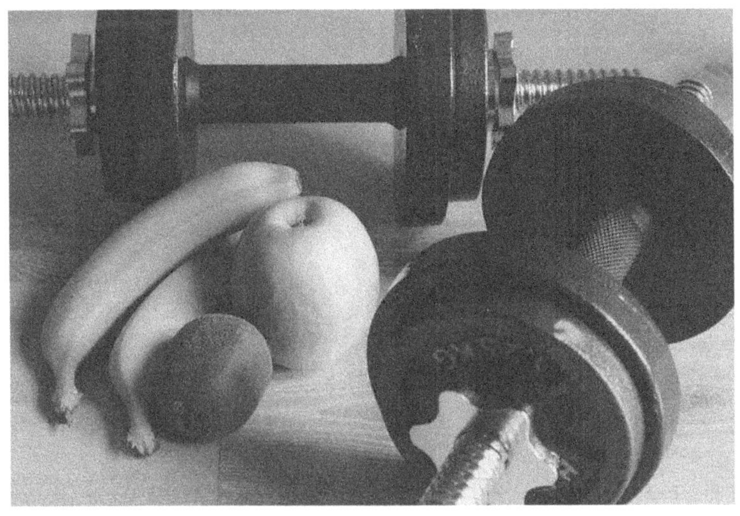

Let me begin by acknowledging that this has been under dispute for a while. But here is the reality; when you have a brief feeding window, you can only have so many meals that need to meet your daily calorie intake. In most instances, you'll concentrate your calories in 1 or 2 consistent meals. This approach has been received well by many bodybuilders compared to having to distribute this same number of calories in up to six meals in a day. Therefore, although it's true that you need a certain proportion of proteins to maintain your muscle mass, you need to realize that you can maintain your muscle mass with intermittent fasting. An increase in the growth hormone makes after 48 hours of fasting makes it possible to maintain your muscle mass without having to take protein shakes or even eat proteins.

## Intermittent Fasting Results in Increased Energy

Although you'll tend to feel sluggish in the initial days of beginning intermittent fasting, your energy levels will not always below. If anything, you'll be surprised how energetic you'll feel because when you fast, your body doesn't rely on the food you're consuming for energy but your energy reserves. This is meant that you'll always feel energetic for a long period.

## Intermittent Fasting Helps to Prevent the Onset of Alzheimer's Disease

Alzheimer's disease is the most popular neurodegenerative disease worldwide. Since this disease has no cure, preventing it is very important. According to a study carried out in rats that also practiced intermittent fasting showed that following intermittent fasting is able to delay the development of Alzheimer's disease. In instances where the disease is already showing, intermittent fasting reduced the severity significantly. Various reports corroborate with this suggesting that a lifestyle intervention that entails short term fasting will improve the symptoms of Alzheimer's disease in nine out of ten patients. Studies that have been conducted in animals show that fasting is capable of protecting against various other neurodegenerative diseases that include Parkinson's disease and Huntington's disease. However, this is not conclusive, hence the need for more studies, especially in human beings.

## Intermittent Fasting Contributes to Improved Physical Fitness

Intermittent fasting has a great impact on your digestive system. Having a short feeding window encourages the proper digestion of food. This encourages healthy and proportional daily intake of food and calories. As you used to your intermittent fasting routine, you'll hardly experience hunger. Although most people argue that intermittent fasting slows down metabolism, but this is just a misconception. If anything, intermittent fasting enhances your metabolism so that it's flexible since your body is able to run on either glucose or fat energy effectively. What this means is that intermittent fasting will enhance your metabolism.

## Intermittent Fasting Will Help in Synchronizing Your Circadian Rhythm as Well as Fight Off Metabolic Diseases

Your circadian rhythm is basically your sleep and wake cycle. That is, this internal and natural system is designed to regulate feelings of wakefulness and sleepiness over 24 hours. According to research, the benefits of following the intermittent fasting lifestyle are that your body is able to adapt to the natural circadian rhythm, which is good for metabolism. Eating just before going to bed has been associated with sleep disturbance as well as weight gain, particularly where it results in acid reflux. This is linked to insulin sensitivity that is really high during the day and low at night—meaning that likely, it's your body that will store most of the glucose consumed at night, leading to weight gain. That's why experts advise that you go to bed early to provide your body with ample time for self-rejuvenation and repair.

## Intermittent Fasting Reduces the Risk of Type 2 Diabetes

The Centre for Disease Control (CDC) estimates that 84.1 million people in the United States are pre-diabetic, a condition that, if left uncontrolled, leads to type 2 diabetes. Intermittent fasting plays an important role in preventing/lowering the risk of type 2 diabetes. This is based on the fact that fasting helps in promoting weight loss that usually has an influence on numerous other factors resulting in a high risk of diabetes. When you lose weight, you'll be insulin sensitive. According to a paper published in the Transnational Research, evidence points to the role of intermittent fasting in reducing the level of insulin as well as blood glucose. This paper further concludes that intermittent fasting will not only help in weight loss but also reducing the risk of diabetes. Adults who practiced intermittent fasting recorded a noticeable decline in diabetes markers like insulin sensitivity in those who are overweight and obese. Thus, it's possible to lower the risk of type 2 diabetes in this demographic since the body will be producing insulin frequently.

Intermittent fasting plays a major role in restoring the secretion of insulin as well as promote the generation of insulin-producing pancreatic beta cells.

## Intermittent Fasting Helps to Fight Off Diseases

When animals are sick, they tend to stop eating until they recover. This is also true for humans. Intermittent fasting is the gateway to your overall well-being since it helps in preventing numerous diseases and medical conditions. Numerous studies have linked intermittent fasting to better overall health. A study published in the World Journal of diabetes has shown that type 2 diabetes patients who practice intermittent fasting on short term experience a reduction in their bodyweight that comes with improved post-meal glucose variability. The other benefits related to this include reduced inflammation, reduced blood pressure, improved glucose circulation, as well as lipid levels that are likely to result in reduced risk of illnesses.

# Intermittent Fasting Helps to Improve Physical Fitness

Besides improved mental performance, intermittent fasting also contributed to improved physical performance. Having an extended fasting period and a short feeding window promotes better digestion resulting in a proportional daily calorie and food intake that is healthy. As you get used to intermittent fasting, you'll most certainly experience hunger at the beginning, but as you fast, your metabolism is enhanced, letting your body run on energy from fats and glucose effectively.

# Intermittent Fasting Helps to Lose Belly Fat and Weight

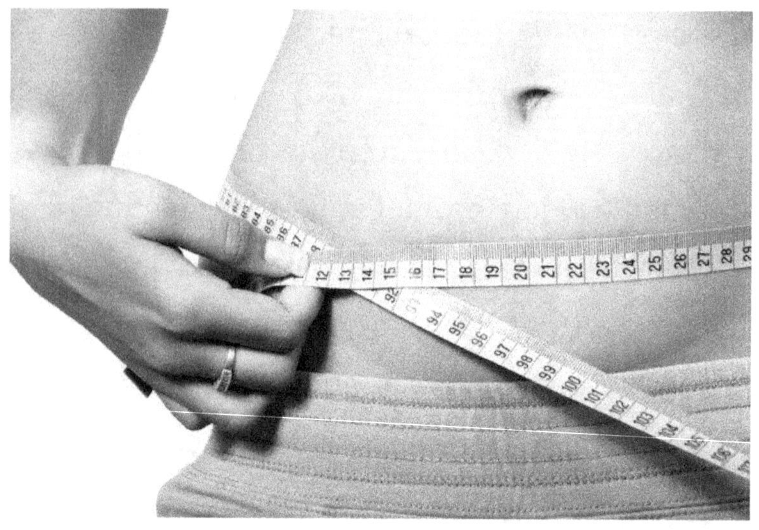

Most people struggle with weight management and weight loss; hence, you may have tried numerous diets before you heard about intermittent fasting. Well, intermittent fasting will drive your weight loss because it lowers your insulin levels. Insulin is the hormone that is responsible for enabling cells to take glucose. When you fast, your body will not have access to glucose for energy. However, when the body enters the fasted state, it breaks down carbohydrates and converts them to glucose that the cells use for energy. Alternatively, they convert it into fat that is then stored. Your insulin level dips when you stop consuming food. This decrease in insulin causes cells to find an alternative source of energy. When you fast repeatedly, you begin to experience loss of weight. This is a shift from what diets are designed to do because most diets get you to avoid certain foods, so when you're done with the diet and must now go back to your normal way of eating, you will end up putting on weight again.

## Intermittent Fasting Promotes Enhanced Cognitive Power

Intermittent fasting promotes your neuronal functionality that tends to decrease as you advance in age. As you grow old, there will be a decline in the number of your dendritic spine, which are the small membranous protrusions that are found on the neuron of the dendrite. The dendritic spines play an important role that involves the transfer of information between nerve cells. Even then, the decline of these spines as a result of aging seriously affects the efficiency of neural processes. Intermittent fasting helps to prevent the reduction of the density of these spines. Findings from a study carried out in rats showed a 38% decrease in the dendritic spines of rates that were on a normal eating pattern. On the contrary, rats that were on the intermittent fasting did not have a significant difference in their dendritic spines. Instead, these rats had an improved learning ability. The calorie reduction that is a result of intermittent fasting enhances the process of neurogenesis that involves the formation of new brain cells while protecting neurons from death. Additionally, fasting also stimulated the production of the Brain-Derived Neurotropic Factor (BDNF), a protein that is associated with the increase in neurogenesis. This is essential in slowing down neuron degenerations as well as the eventual cell aging. Neurogenesis also promotes functional recovery and healing of any injuries to the spinal cord in animals regardless of whether intermittent fasting is introduced after or before the injury.

## Intermittent Fasting Minimizes the Risk of Cancer

Intermittent fasting helps in slowing down the development as well as the progression of malignant tumors. Rats that were transplanted with a cancer cell line and subjected to intermittent fasting survived longer than those that were free-fed. After ten days, half of the rats that were subjected to intermittent fasting were alive. On the contrary, only 12.5% of the rats in the control group survived. In yet another study involving middle ages rats that were introduced to intermittent fasting and put under observation for four months, there was a notable reduction in the incidence of lymphoma. Although 30% of the mice in the control group got ill, none of those that were on intermittent fasting became cancerous. Intermittent fasting also saw a decline in the development of pre-neoplastic liver surgery and liver nodule, which are usually a result of carcinogenic substances. The rats that ate intermittently also had improved antioxidant activity that results in a reduction in the development of the free harmful radicals within mitochondria. It's important to note that the anti-tumor effect is not a product of calorie reduction because both groups consumed an equal amount of calories.

## Intermittent Fasting Enhances Better Heart Health

A study that was done among participants who were non-obese to determine the benefits of practicing intermittent fasting. The findings of the study reveal a decline in triglyceride in men. On the other hand, there was an increase in the levels of good HDL cholesterol in women. This change was recorded 22 days after the participants had taken part in the study. This change was mainly associated with a 4% degradation in body fat. There was an even better improvement in people who were obese as they were able to shed off an average of 5.6 kilograms within eight weeks of intermittent fasting. This was translated to a 21% decline in the levels of cholesterol, a 25% decline in the LDL cholesterol levels, and a 32% decrease in the level of triglycerides. In a similar manner, there was a notable drop in the systolic blood pressure from 124mmHg to 116 mmHg. Besides the reduction in body weight, intermittent fasting will also prompt stress resistance that produces a cardioprotective effect. Studies carried out in mice also show that when there is a heart attack, the area that is affected is much smaller in mice that were subject to intermittent fasting compare to the mice that were normally fed. Moreover, four times fewer did heart muscles die in mice that were fed intermittently.

# Intermittent Fasting Contributes to Extending Your Lifespan and Longevity

During intermittent fasting, your body experiences calorie restriction as a result of a shortened feeding window and a longer fasting window. Calorie restriction has the potential of increasing your lifespan considerably. Fasting has also been found to increase the lifespan of various organisms that include yeast and worms. While this pattern of eating's main focus is not calorie restriction, intermittent fasting results in reduced calorie consumption by up to 30%. This promotes enhanced insulin sensitivity a decline in the damage of free radicals and damage to the cellular components that include proteins and DNA, a decrease in the blood pressure as well as heart rate, a decline in the incidence of induced as well as spontaneous tumors and improved resistance to neurodegenerative diseases. Intermittent fasting is a great alternative to calorie restriction that produces a similar effect in the extension of your lifespan and on the aging process in general. Young rats that were subjected to fasting recorded a longer lifespan that exceeded their average lifespan by several months. This same effect is experienced in human beings because fasting sends your body into stress as a result of calorie withdrawal. This is followed by the release of chemicals that cushion you from the effects of fasting. It also helps to fix depression and anxiety. These chemicals also help the body to develop resistance to stress that eventually slows down the aging process.

# Chapter 5:

# Intermittent Fasting and Autophagy

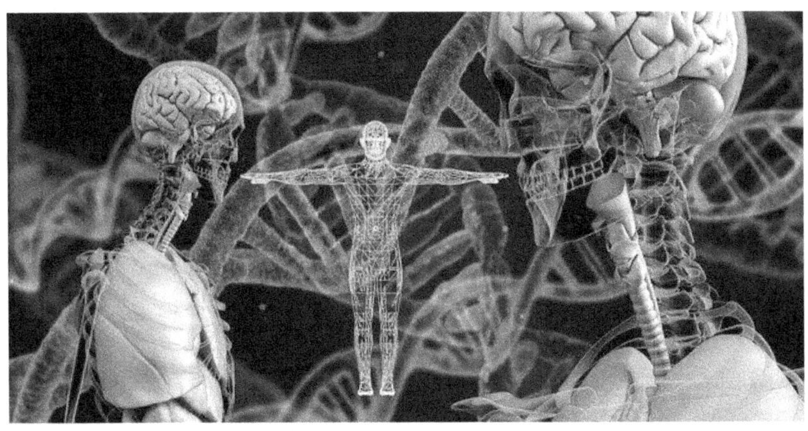

You cannot talk about intermittent fasting without talking about autophagy. So, what is autophagy? Autophagy refers to the process through which the body gets rid of old cells in a process that involves the regeneration of newer, healthier cells. Autophagy is a term that comes from two words: auto, which means self, and phagy, which means to eat. Therefore, autophagy is the process of self-eating—a self-preservation mechanism that allows your body to eliminate any dysfunctional cells even as it recycles some of the parts of these cells in order to facilitate cellular cleaning and repair.

A Belgian scientist, Christian de Duve, was the first person to come up with the term autophagy following a study he was doing on the roles of glucagon and lysosomes in cell degeneration. This was followed by research on autophagy by researchers, with most of them focusing on cellular autophagy. However, the challenge was that there was scanty information on the importance of this process not just to the human body but the overall well-being as well.

Things took a new twist in 1983 when Yoshinori Ohsumi discovered the gene that played an important role in regulating autophagy in yeast. This was a significant breakthrough because he found that the yeast cells that did not have the said gene did not undergo autophagy. Moreover, they could also not go through the regeneration process. This discovery earned Ohsumi a Nobel Prize in 2016. Among the greatest lessons from Ohsumi's discovery is the manner in which cells respond to a deficiency in nutrients, cellular injuries, an increase in the levels of stress as well as deprivation of energy through an increase in the rate of cellular autophagy. However, when stress is eliminated, the process of autophagy goes back to maintenance mode, which is basically the normal rate. There's a need to carry out more studies to have a better understanding of the autophagy process and its anti-aging properties. This is because it is widely believed that by promoting the process of cell regeneration, autophagy has the capacity to increase your lifespan.

## The Process of Autophagy

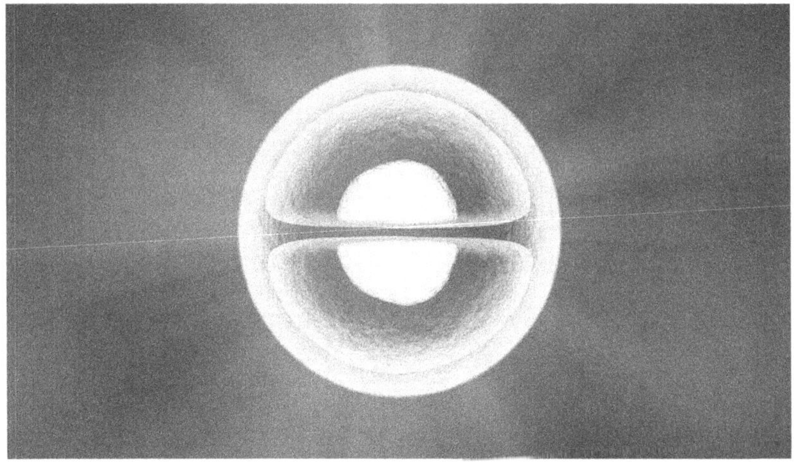

The main goal of the autophagy process is self-regulation and removal of debris, ensuring optimal smooth functioning. This means that it cleans and recycles at the same time. The autophagy process also enhances survival and adaptation as a response to the stressors and toxins that will accumulate inside the cells over time, making them become junky and old, hence requiring a replacement. During this process, both cellular and sub-cellular debris are eliminated. This process occurs when the old cells are sent to the lysosome, which is a special organelle with enzymes that have the ability to degrade proteins. When autophagy takes place, the subcellular parts that are damaged, as well as the unused proteins are isolated for destruction before they can be sent to lysosomes for final processing.

## Forms of Autophagy

There are three different types of autophagy—namely, chaperone-mediated autophagy, macroautophagy, and microautophagy. However, the most common of these three is macroautophagy, which is an evolutionary conserved catabolic process involving the formation of vesicles/autophagosomes that engulf macromolecules and cellular organelles.

# Chaperone-Mediated Autophagy

In this form of autophagy, the cell makes use of chaperone proteins such as Hsc-70 found in the lysosomal membrane. These proteins will bind on the unwanted protein molecules found in the cell, forming a chaperone complex/substrate. This molecule will then attach onto the wall of the lysosome, making room for the protein molecules to enter the lysosome for disintegration.

# Macro-Autophagy

This autophagy process involves the transportation of all the waste material inside a cell via an autophagosome, which is basically a double membrane-bound vesicle into the lysosome. The autophagosome then fuses with the lysosome, effectively emptying all the content and thus creating room for the processing of the waste materials.

# Micro-Autophagy

During micro-autophagy, cellular waste, which is supposed to be digested, is wiped out by the lysosomes either by developing cellular protrusions or through the inward folding of a part of the lysosomal membrane.

Although the mechanism is different, the three autophagy processes involve non-selective as well as selective degradation methods that are reliant on organelles or molecules that need to be broken down or recycled. Eventually, each of the cellular components that need to be degraded is mopped from the lysosome, followed by conversion into micro molecules such as glucose, fatty acids, nucleotides, and amino acids. The cell reuses these micro molecules to form larger molecules and new organelles. Such autophagy processes rejuvenate your body's cells, making you feel better, younger, and healthier.

# What Does It Take to Activate Autophagy?

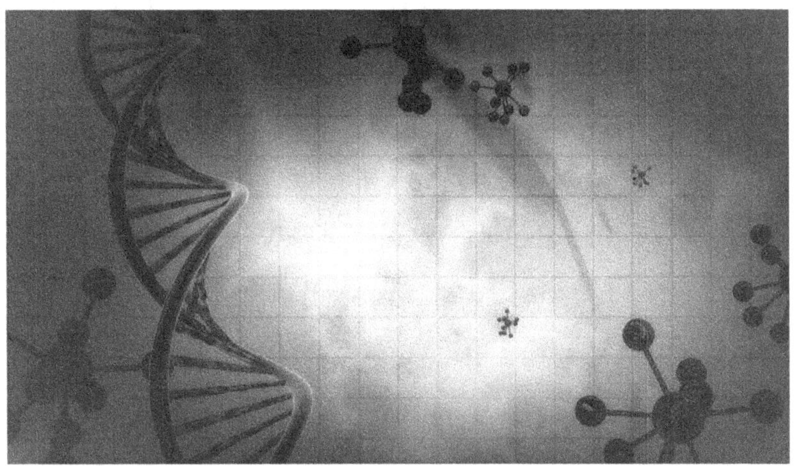

Although everyone wants to tap into the benefits of autophagy, especially longevity, you need to know that not all forms of intermittent fasting are able to activate autophagy. In fact, autophagy is not activated the moment you begin intermittent fasting. It kicks in after hours of fasting. To be more precise, autophagy is mainly activated by nutrient deprivation along with numerous other factors such as your level of activity and the percentage of your body fat. Principally, autophagy depends on the effort you're willing to put in so as to get your body to activate autophagy. Whenever the level of nutrients such as amino acids, glucose, and calories are low, this necessitates autophagy. The reason for this is simple; the body is not motivated to seek alternative energy from alternative sources like body tissues and fat stores. Even then, this can happen under the right conditions. When the body has sufficient nutrients, AMPK and mTOR receive the signal. These cells decide whether they will promote growth or simply switch to intermittent fasting. Other factors that have an impact on autophagy include growth factors such as IGF-1, mechanical muscle stimuli, and insulin.

In general, you need to fast for between 48 to 72 hours in order to activate autophagy. Incidentally, this is the time it also takes for the body to undergo ketosis, where it produces ketones. Although there's no proper way of determining the rate of autophagy, especially in humans, it can be estimated by looking at the glucose ketone index as well as the insulin to glucose ratio. When this ratio is low, various things happen, which include ketogenesis, gluconeogenesis, fat oxidation, and the breakdown of nutrients. The duration needed for autophagy to kick will be determined by your body nutrients, glucose, amino acids, and the presence of nutrients in your ketones. This means that if your body is conditioned not to consume excess fat and protein daily, it will be faster to enter autophagy than someone who has to burn many calories in the initial stages.

# Benefits of Autophagy

One of the reasons why people can't stop talking about autophagy is because of the numerous benefits it offers. As various metabolic activities take place, the result is cellular damage, especially to the human body. The rate of the occurrence of cellular damage is aggravated by a poor diet, exposure to radiation, and stress, among other things. Thus, autophagy helps to clean out the old and damaged cells that are no longer active. This process helps to purge the body from pathogens that cause diseases. It also gives rise to a number of benefits that include the following:

# Decreases the Risk of Cell Death

In certain instances, the cells in your body may be degraded so much that they can longer be regenerated or replaced, and the only option left is cell death that is also referred to as apoptosis. This is not good because the cells that are spared when cell death occurs are usually irreparable, so losing them means a total loss. Autophagy comes in to prevent such a scenario as well as prevent diseases that are associated with cell death.

## Extends Lifespan

While there are a number of techniques and methods that guarantee you an improvement of health along with other benefits, autophagy is the most outstanding in this respect. Since cells are the building blocks of life and autophagy plays a critical role in eliminating waste from the cells, the removal of substances that are perceived to be toxic will help to promote the cell metabolic efficiency. The cellular regeneration and degeneration that is triggered by autophagy will help you in staying more youthful than you are. This is especially great for your skin that is often exposed to harsh elements and pollutants, resulting in wrinkles as well as a decline in your skin quality.

## Regulates Inflammation

The process of autophagy can either improve or minimize your immune response by preventing or promoting inflammation. When there is an invade, autophagy will boost inflammation by alerting your immune system to attack. It can also decrease inflammation by eliminating all the signals that trigger it.

## Improves Your Skin

The skin is the largest organ in the body, but it is prone to damage from various factors like air pollution, adverse weather, chemicals, sunshine, heat, and light, among other things. These make it grow old faster. When autophagy is activated, it helps in the replacement of the old cells with new ones while at the same time repairing the old cells. This is good, as the skin cells contribute to getting rid of bacteria that infiltrate the body; hence, you have to energize them for them to be active.

## Helps to Improve Metabolism

Autophagy helps in boosting your body's metabolism. This is achieved through the regeneration and replacement of the important cells that are related to your metabolism, like mitochondria. This affects the performance of your muscles, effectively promoting the development of your muscle mass and the growth of your cells. This also prevents any stress that is linked to injuries to the muscles.

# Protects from Neurodegenerative Disorders

Autophagy plays an important role in the prevention of the onset of some of the neurodegenerative diseases like Alzheimer's diseases, Parkinson's disease, and dementia, among others. These diseases are known to thrive with an accumulation of old and toxic neurons that pile in specific areas in the brain before they begin spreading to the surrounding areas. This means that autophagy has the capability of replacing parts of the useless neuron before they regenerate new ones.

# Combats Infectious Diseases

Autophagy helps to swing your immune system into action. This process can help to eliminate some microbes like mycobacterium tuberculosis as well as other deadly viruses such as HIV from your body cells. Autophagy will take care of the toxins that come about because of the infections.

## Helps to Strengthen the Immunity System

When activated, autophagy helps in keeping your body from possible infections through the removal of toxins from the cells. This process is also responsible for the destruction of harmful microbes through the promotion of inflammation on the cells and fighting diseases. Cellular inflammation will enhance the immune system of the cells when there is an impending attack from various diseases. Autophagy prompts inflammation by making the proteins to work actively by starving them of nutrients. This initiates a requisite immune response that fights diseases and infections.

## Prevents the Onset of Cancer

One of the reasons why autophagy continues to draw the attention of the medical world is because of its ability to prevent the onset of cancer. Autophagy has been found to inhibit or prevent the development of early stages of cancer. This is linked to the fact that cancer is a disease that results from cellular disorders. Thus, the process of autophagy helps to prevent such disorders through the regulation of damage response that is caused by the promotion of cellular inflammation, DNA, and regulation of genome instability.

## Helps the Body to Deal with Stress

The process of autophagy has been found to be helpful in the treatment as well as prevention of some psychiatric conditions such as depression and schizophrenia.

Despite all the benefits discussed above, you must keep in mind that autophagy also presents a number of negative side effects, for instance, it could provide a conducive atmosphere for certain bacteria such as Brucella, Coxiella, and Bartonella to not only divide but also multiply. When this happens, you'll end up with an overgrowth of bacteria. Moreover, recent studies have cast doubt on the ability of autophagy to hinder the multiplication of cancer cells. The studies suggest that autophagy could, in fact, promote the multiplication of cancer, causing cells. As such, autophagy is seen as a strong preventative measure as opposed to a treatment.

# Chapter 6:

# Intermittent Fasting for Women

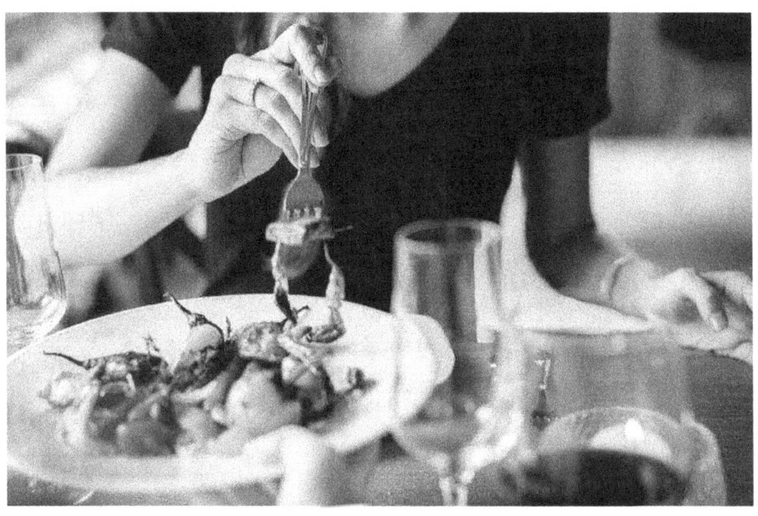

The female body responds to calorie deprivation differently than the male body. As such, women who practice intermittent fasting experience a host of changes in their bodies. These changes are linked to hormonal imbalance, and they include missed menstrual periods, metabolic disturbances, and for some, menopause that kicks in early. In this chapter, we take a closer look at intermittent fasting in women and what women need to do to minimize the undesirable effects.

## Effects of Intermittent Fasting in Women

Women must approach intermittent fasting with caution because failure to do so can result in adverse effects. A woman's body is extremely sensitive to the signals of starvation. This means whenever the body senses starvation, it'll raise the production of the two hunger hormones known as leptin and ghrelin. Consequently, when women experience hunger, it's actually because of the increased production of hunger hormones. This is a survival mechanism for the female body as it seeks to offer protection for a potential fetus. This will happen even when you're not pregnant.

On the other hand, restricting calories could also result in the inhibition of the production of female sex hormones. This can lead to infertility in some women, while others could experience irregular periods, halted ovulation, and hormonal imbalances. This could affect your menstruation and eventually cause the ovaries to shrink. Some women who practice intermittent fasting may also end up with disordered eating manifesting through eating disorders such as anorexia and binge eating.

Because of all these reasons, women who desire to practice intermittent fasting mist not focus on calorie restriction but the health and wellness angle. Otherwise, you will end up with a number of changes that you cannot bear and can hamper the normal optimal functioning of your body. Some of the common changes you can expect when you take on intermittent fasting include the following:

## Hormonal Imbalance

It's not unusual for women who are practicing intermittent fasting for the first time to experience hormonal imbalances. After all, women are at one point or the other experiencing hormonal imbalances. Even then, you must keep in mind that when you introduce intermittent fasting, this could evolve to issues associated with genetics. Some of the concerns associated with hormonal imbalance during intermittent fasting include the irregular length of the menstrual period, irregular menstruation, irregular strength of your flow, and blemishes that are difficult to clear as well as changes in the color of your skin.

## Emotional Instability

Hormonal imbalance comes along with emotional instability. You may experience periods of excitement, followed by periods of sadness. However, this doesn't go on for long and should ease up as you get used to your intermittent fasting schedule.

## Excessive Fatigue

A reduction in the number of calories you consume on a given day comes with two most pronounced side effects that are fatigue and muscle weakness. These effects are compounded by the fact that the female body mostly depends on glucose from food than stored fat for energy. While these effects will be minimal as time goes by and even disappear, they make the adaptation as well as transition to intermittent fasting somewhat difficult.

# How to Practice Intermittent Fasting Safely as a Woman

Despite the changes that you're bound to go through when practicing intermittent fasting, you can still come up with a safer way of doing intermittent fasting to minimize the negative effects and get the most out of practice. Here are some guidelines to help you practice intermittent fasting safely as a woman:

## Start Slowly and Adjust Accordingly

Regardless of the intermittent fasting plan that you decide to start with, make sure that start slowly and gradually increases the hours of fasting as your body gets used to it. You can begin by limiting your consumption of carbs and instead focus on foods that are high in healthy fat and proteins.

## Assess Your Levels of Stress

Fasting puts stress on your body with the potential of causing negative effects. Therefore, when you notice some adverse signs of hormonal imbalance at the beginning of intermittent fasting, make a point of stopping or modifying your intermittent fasting plan. Modifying your plan could mean increasing your feeding window as you shorten the fasting window.

## Eat Fewer Calories

If you're embracing intermittent fasting in order to shed off some weight, you need to make sure that your overall calorie consumption is less than what you need to maintain your current weight. This will help you to shed off excessive weight.

Overall, women who follow a shorted fasting window of between 12 and 14 hours have reported better results.

# Benefits of Intermittent Fasting for Women

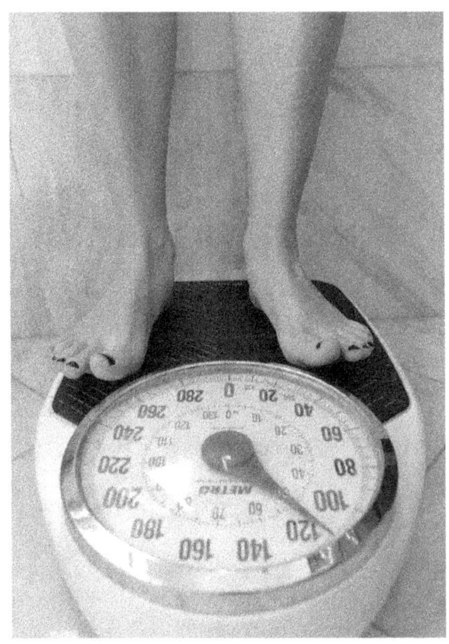

One of the most common benefits of intermittent fasting among women is weight loss. However, women who practice intermittent fasting enjoy numerous other benefits that include the following:

## Improved Metabolic Health

Postmenopausal women have a high risk of experiencing cardiovascular diseases. This is attributed to the increase in LDL cholesterol, belly fats as well as high triglyceride levels. High levels of insulin and glucose are also considered to have an impact. Studies show that women who fast have a notable improvement in their metabolic health as these symptoms lessen, thereby removing the risk of cardiovascular diseases.

## Reproductive Health Benefits

Various studies have associated intermittent fasting for women to reproductive health benefits. Several health conditions relating to endocrine dysfunction in women, such as Polycystic ovarian syndrome (PCOS), obesity, and metabolic syndrome, could be improved by practicing intermittent fasting. One study carried out among women who had polycystic ovarian syndrome established that there was a decrease in stress neurohormone levels, which had a positive effect on mental and physical health. Yet another study found that short term restriction of calories resulted in an increase in the luteinizing hormone, particularly in women who had PCOS. This hormone is produced in the pituitary glance and plays an important role in ensuring healthy patterns of ovulation. This is suitable, taking into account hormone balancing, as it's also a fertility marker.

# Mental Health Benefits

Statistics from the World Health Organization (WHO) indicate that women have a higher percentage of mental health disorders, particularly depression and stress. One of the reasons for this trend is that the major stressor is food. The outer appearance and weight have been made to look like something that one needs to fix constantly. Unfortunately, this also affects how women feel about themselves, thus creating so many insecurities. Intermittent fasting will help you to tap into the inherent health and simplify the mental burden, so you don't have to think about what to eat. It will also help you to address hormonal instability during menopause that has been associated with emotional pressure tension, depression, and anxiety. Intermittent fasting will help to improve your self-esteem and mental status, reduce anxiety and depression, and promote social functioning.

# Musculoskeletal Health Benefits

Chronic pain disorders tend to be on the rise in women who are in their 40s. They include osteoporosis, arthritis, chronic back pain, and fibromyalgia, among others.

Intermittent fasting helps in supporting musculoskeletal conditions in women. One study showed the effect of the parathyroid hormone in improving bone health as well as cases of rheumatoid arthritis. Fasting will also improve the symptoms of intestinal permeability that effectively leads to decreased food intolerance. This also results in a reduction in the inflammatory markers as well as the prevention of the vicious circle of inflammation that includes rheumatoid arthritis. Weight loss from intermittent fasting will also support musculoskeletal health since fasting supports the normalization of hormones that determine your weight; thus, fasting is a great way of remedying musculoskeletal health.

The other benefits of intermittent fasting include more energy, sustainable weight loss, an increase in the lean muscle mass, reduced inflammation, reduced oxidative stress, an increase in cell stress response, an increase in the production of neurotrophic growth factors and improved insulin sensitivity. Intermittent fasting is an excellent way of making lifestyle changes to your eating pattern as well as taking charge of your health. This makes it ideal for women who have struggled with weight loss and other related issues for long.

# Disadvantages of Intermittent Fasting for Women

In spite of all the benefits discussed above, intermittent fasting also presents a number of disadvantages in different categories of women. Some of the disadvantages of intermittent fasting include the following:

- Some women find it difficult to sleep because of the hormonal imbalance resulting from fasting.

- You may end up experiencing fertility issues. This is why it is important that you stop intermittent fasting whenever you experience something that is out of the ordinary.

- For some women, the ovaries could shrink, and this can be a huge disadvantage, especially in women of childbearing age.

- You could also experience metabolic stress, irregular periods, and anxiety—all of which are a cause for concern.

Since hormones are mostly interconnected in the

functionality, destabilizing one hormone is likely to have a negative effect on all the other hormones. This should not be a reason to give up intermittent fasting. Rather, you can use fasting to complement a healthy diet and lifestyle.

## Intermittent Fasting in Post-Menopausal Women

Menopause is not often a great time for most women because of the host of changes that they experience that are out of their control. This includes hot flashes, mood swings, cravings, interrupted sleep, and low self-esteem, among others. For most women dealing with some of these symptoms can be extremely overwhelming. However, studies point to intermittent fasting to be a great solution that is producing great results. For instance, women who are post-menopausal have been shown to lose twice as much weight as women who are yet to attain menopause. This is linked to better diet adherence. According to these findings, intermittent fasting is seen as being beneficial for women who have already attained menopause.

Intermittent fasting is a great solution to losing belly fat and the prevention of weight gain both during and post-menopause. Fasting intermittently will also help to lower the risk of diabetes by reducing blood cholesterol and blood pressure while enhancing insulin resistance. Even then, you need also to understand that the fact that intermittent fasting may have worked for someone else doesn't mean that it will also work for you. The reason for this is simple. Different people will respond differently to different intermittent fasting methods. Therefore, it's up to you to identify the intermittent fasting method that suits you in terms of your needs and lifestyle. Remember, your body is highly sensitive to changes during menopause. Therefore, consider getting into intermittent fasting gradually so that you get used to your fasting window until you get comfortable as opposed to starting with fasting for long hours. You can also test to determine if taking fluids only during your fasting window will increase or ease your menopause symptoms. Should you notice that the symptoms are increasing, then you must stop right away, take a break before you consider trying another intermittent fasting method. Here are some tips for getting into intermittent fasting after menopause safely:

- Begin by fasting for 12 hours and a feeding period of 12 hours.

- Increase the fasting window gradually as you get comfortable until you get to fast for 16 hours with a feeding window of 4 hours.

- Avoid the temptation of extreme fasting beyond the 16-hour window.

- Make sure you're well-hydrated by consuming a lot of fluids that are free of calories when fasting.

- You can introduce gentle exercises as you pay attention to the way your body will respond.

## How Intermittent Fasting Affects Fertility

Various studies done in worms and mice suggest that intermittent fasting is able to help in extending fertility in women. This is based on the understanding that when you restrict the consumption of food, the quality of eggs improves a great deal. This is because both the quantity and quality of eggs is linked to aging. A study conducted in adult female mice found that was under intermittent fasting found that the eggs from the mice that experienced calorie restriction were more likely to develop into fertilized embryos. Research also shows that as little as a 5 to 10 percent drop in weight has significant benefits in the improvement of psychological outcomes, reproductive features, and metabolic features.

# Chapter 7:

# Foods and Drinks Included in the Intermittent Fasting Plan

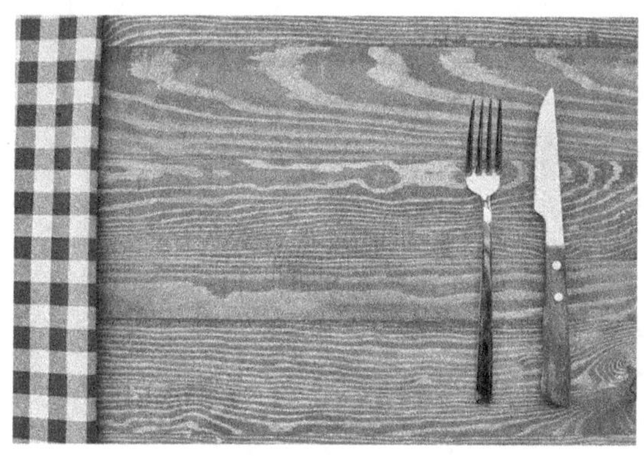

Unlike most diets that are specific about the types of food you should eat and in what proportion, intermittent fasting takes a different approach—that is, it's not strict on the foods you should eat; rather, you're free to eat whatever you want, but it emphasizes clean eating. The reason for this is simple; if you are battling weight, chances are it took time to get to where you are. Therefore, in the same manner, it'll take time before you shake off the excessive weight. This means that the fact that you're fasting doesn't mean that you can throw down some junk food when the feeding window comes and expect to get results.

## Foods to Eat During Intermittent Fasting

Intermittent fasting eventually results in the form of calorie restriction because of the shortened feeding duration. I mean, you can only eat so much. As such, if you don't plan your meals well, chances are you'll end up being nutrient deficient. Therefore, it is imperative that you make the right food choices so that you get enough nutrients and keep your blood sugar stable. If you don't know what foods you can eat and drink, you can get some inspiration from the following:

## Minimally Processed Grains

Most diets will omit carbohydrates because they are responsible for weight gain. Well, it's important to perceive the importance of carbohydrates as part of your nutrition and not an enemy for your ambition to lose weight. The fact that you spent most of the hours fasting, you must be strategic when it comes to getting your calories without being too full. You can consider including minimally processed grains as these are a quick source of fuel because they can be digested fast. Minimally processed grains are particularly great if you like to train because you get energy almost instantly.

## Raspberries

The fact that you're fasting means that you need foods that are high in fiber to help in maintaining regular bowel movement as well as help you to feel fuller for longer. Interestingly, most dietary guidelines miss out on this. It has been observed that less than 10% of western populations consume sufficient amounts of whole fruits. Raspberries are a great choice when you're fasting because they're high in fiber. A single cup of raspberries will give you about 8 grams of fiber that is able to carry you through your fasting window.

## Wild-Caught Salmon

This fish is mostly consumed across the blue zones of the five regions of Latin America, Asia, Europe, and the U.S. that are known for dietary and lifestyle choices that are linked to extreme longevity. Wild-caught salmon contains high levels of omega 3 fatty acids EPA and DHA that are also great in boosting cognitive abilities.

## Seitan

It's a good idea that you incorporate plant-based proteins into your diet like seitan. This protein offers you amazing anti-aging properties in your diet to complement your intermittent fasting. This is a good alternative considering the recommendation by the EAT-Lancet commission that you should consume animal proteins in smaller quantities. In fact, red meat has been linked to an increase in mortality. Seitan offers the versatility of preparation as you can dip it, bake it, or even batter it in your favorite sauces.

## Hummus

This is another great source of plant protein that will greatly boost your nutritional value of certain staples like sandwiches. Although you can take the adventurous path and make your own, the secret to the best recipe is ample garlic, as well as tahini.

# Soybeans

Soybeans are not only a great choice because they help you stay fuller for longer but also have anti-aging properties. They contain an active compound known as isoflavones, which promote anti-aging, in addition to having the ability to hinder UVB induced cell damage. Including soybeans in your meals during intermittent fasting will certainly compliment the benefits you derive from the autophagy process.

# Potatoes

Potatoes compare to bread by the mere fact that they are easy to digest with very little effort. Potatoes also make a perfect post work out snack when you pair them with a great source of protein because you can be sure to refuel the muscles better. One other factor that makes potatoes a great choice is because when cooled, potatoes go on to form a resistant starch that it plays a crucial role in fueling the good bacteria that is found in the gut.

# Lentils

This is another excellent source of plant proteins that are

also packed with fiber. Lentils can give you at least 32% of your daily recommended fiber intake. Additionally, lentils are also a great source of iron, taking up at about 15% of your daily needs. This is especially great for women who are active and are practicing intermittent fasting.

## Milk-Fortified with Vitamin D

An average adult should take at least 1,000 milligrams of calcium per day. This translated to about 3 cups of milk daily. When you practice intermittent fasting, the short feeding window means a reduced opportunity to take as much milk as you should. This means that you must make a point of prioritizing your consumption of foods that are rich in calcium. Milk fortified with vitamin D is an excellent choice because it will enhance the consumption of calcium, thereby helping to keep your bones strong. You can add milk to smoothies and cereal or simply take it along with your meals.

## Multivitamins

The fact that your nutrition during intermittent fasting is

based on the amount of time you have to eat means you must make extremely good choices and opt for healthy meal considerations. This will help to avoid vitamin deficiencies that may be a result of shorter feeding hours. Therefore, make sure you include plenty of fruits and vegetables so that you have a sufficient intake of vitamins.

## Other Food Options

There are many other food options that you can include in your diet during intermittent fasting. They include olives, blueberries, papaya, nuts, ghee, avocado, cruciferous vegetables, eggs, probiotics, and whole grains, among others. Most importantly, before making any changes to your diet significantly, it's important that you speak with a nutritionist or a health professional to make sure you're making the right strides.

## Drinks to Take During Intermittent Fasting

One of the fears of most people who want to adopt the intermittent fasting lifestyle having to go for long hours without food and drink. Even then, intermittent fasting is quite flexible because you can be able to drink up fluids that do not contain any calories throughout the fasting window. Here are some of the drinks that you are allowed to take throughout your intermittent fasting period:

## Black Coffee

There's a common misconception that taking coffee during intermittent fasting will break your fast. This is not true. In fact, studies have shown that consuming caffeine when you're fasting will actually increase your metabolism that will promote the loss of weight. Black coffee is also known to help in suppressing appetite, making it a great choice because it will help you to get through your fast and make it more manageable. However, you must not add any syrups, candied flavorings, or even cream, as all these have the potential of breaking your fast because they contain calories. Most importantly, you should also not go overboard with the coffee because taking too much coffee will make you feel weak, jittery, and anxious, especially when you're sensitive to caffeine. Moreover, too much coffee may also interrupt your sleep patterns and the quality of your sleep. Remember, taking coffee on an empty stomach will result in fast assimilation into the bloodstream compared to taking coffee alongside meals. Thus, you can limit your intake to about two cups that is equivalent to 400mg of caffeine.

## Water

Staying well-hydrated is important when you need to maintain a healthy system. Drinking water does in no way break your fast. In fact, water is one of the best drinks you can take when fasting because it is full of minerals that are important in the restoration of electrolyte and mineral balance. When you abstain from food for 12-16 hours, your body will turn to the glycogen that is stored in the liver. Moreover, you'll also lose a lot of fluid and electrolytes as the stored energy is being broken down into glucose. This means that drinking 8 glasses of water shall promote the smooth flow of blood and cognition while preventing dehydration. Taking water also goes a long way in promoting your joint and muscle support. Ideally, you should drink at least half of your body weight but in terms of ounces. This is in addition to the other beverages that you'll be consuming.

Taking water also helps you to deal with hunger as it helps you feel full, making it a lot easier to follow your intermittent fasting protocol to the latter with little or no struggle. Taking water will also help in lubricating joints, promote proper bowel movement, and regulate your body temperature. Water also plays a crucial role in transporting oxygen and other nutrients to your cells while at the same time flushing out waste. You can take flavored, plain or carbonated water as long as it's not sweetened. Taking plain water is not usually easy, so you can consider carbonated or flavored water. However, pay attention to the labels on the water just to be sure that it has not been sweetened. Remember, even non-calorie sweeteners like stevia will kick-start your craving for sugar, which will make it difficult for you to stick to your intermittent fasting plan.

## Apple Cider Vinegar

Diluting a small portion of apple cider vinegar in the water will certainly not break your fast. A study that was published in the Journal of Medicinal Food established that apple cider vinegar is able to promote positive metabolic change that helps in promoting weight loss.

Taking apple cider vinegar every day will also contribute to a reduction in your total cholesterol, triglycerides, and LDL levels. This is in addition to lowering your blood sugar levels and improving the digestion process. Even then, avoid the temptation of taking undiluted apple cider vinegar because the acetic acid in it is potent and could damage your teeth's caramel.

## Tea

Just like coffee, taking tea when you're on an intermittent fast won't break your fast. In fact, tea is a great choice of beverage to take when fasting as long as you don't sweeten with sugar or other sweeteners. You should also not add cream. You can try different variations of tea, such as green tea that is packed with powerful antioxidants that will help in burning calories. Other alternatives to tea include chamomile tea, purple tea, and herbal tea, among others. While taking unsweetened tea may be difficult in the beginning, it will get better over time. You will be surprised that this can eventually become a part of your lifestyle.

There are certain drinks that you should avoid taking

during intermittent fasting because even though they may seem to be calorie-free, they will break your fast. A good example is diet soda because it doesn't have any carbohydrates, sugar, or calories. Diet soda may appeal to you as a perfect alternative to taking water, but it's packed with artificial sweeteners that can increase your craving for sugar as well as insulin resistance. This will eventually increase your risk of developing diabetes, making it even more difficult to achieve weight loss. You should also avoid taking all kinds of juices during intermittent fasting because they contain sugar, vitamins, and minerals that will break your fast. However, you may take juices during your feeding window. Alcohol is also a no go zone when you're fasting because it will be absorbed in your bloodstream quickly, given that you will have abstained from food for several hours. As a result, you could end up with dehydration and increased intoxication.

# Chapter 8: Potential Risk of Intermittent Fasting

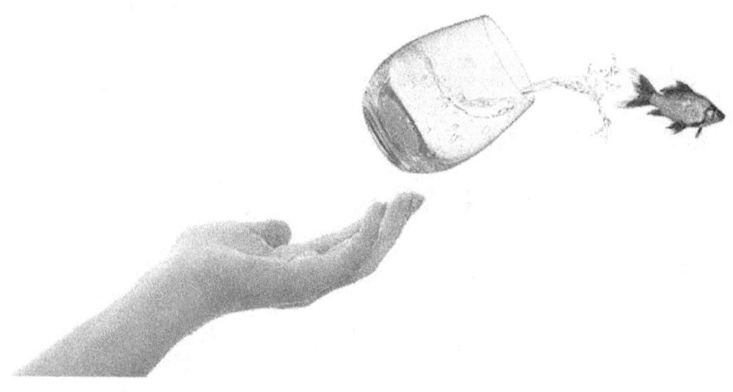

Many people, including celebrities, swear by intermittent fasting obviously because of the many benefits that it offers. However, this eating pattern can pose certain risks when not followed properly or when followed by individuals who shouldn't like expectant women, nursing mothers, people below the age of 18, and those who have previously battled eating disorders. Besides, it has also been argued that most of the studies on intermittent fasting have been done on animals, hence the need for more studies in human beings to validate those studies.

If you're going to practice intermittent fasting and are taking medications, you must begin by consulting the doctor. You need to be certain that fasting will in no way interfere with the effectiveness of your medication. Moreover, if you're the kind of person who has a tight schedule, you must give yourself time to get used to intermittent fasting by beginning with a few hours of fasting while you extend your fasting window gradually. Most importantly, make sure you stick to a nutritious diet and while staying well-hydrated.

The impact of intermittent fasting on your lifestyle cannot be underestimated. However, most people don't stop to think about the potential risks of intermittent fasting before getting into it, yet these risks have a huge impact on whether you will succeed with intermittent fasting or not. Although it is argued that you can easily make intermittent fasting a part of your lifestyle, this can apply to certain intermittent fasting methods. In fact, one of the issues that keep on coming up about intermittent fasting is sustainability.

While most people feel good following an intermittent

fasting lifestyle, it becomes a struggle when you have to stick with it in the long term. This is particularly tricky when you have to fit the eating and fasting cycles in your social and work life. This is especially difficult if you have to work for long hours, go to bed late and wake up early. It's equally difficult if your schedule lacks consistency because you will end up being frustrated for not being able to keep up. For some people, it may be that you just jumped into the intermittent fasting bandwagon without proper preparation, so you end up with a mind-body disconnect making it difficult to establish an overall healthy diet in the long term.

That is why it is important that you begin by talking to your physician before you can begin following any of the intermittent fasting patterns. People who have health complications, an existing medical condition, or are over 65 are more susceptible to the risks of intermittent fasting. If you're taking any medication, you also need to choose an intermittent fasting pattern that is built around the time when you eat. Some of the potential risks of intermittent fasting include the following:

# You Might Overeat

Most people fall for the temptation of overeating on their non-fasting days. This is dangerous because you will most likely end up with a net calorie surplus that will result in weight gain. The challenge could be that fasting will trigger binge eating. A study carried out in 2015 found that intermittent fasting increased the levels of the stress hormone known as cortisol. This eventually results in an increase in cravings. If you're used to eating three meals practicing intermittent fasting can cause stress. This is bad for a stress eater, make sure you engage in activities that lower your cortisol levels like listening to music or meditating. You also must make sure you fill up nutritious and satiating foods.

# You Might Feel Lethargic

Don't be surprised when you start feeling groggy when you start intermittent fasting for the first time. The reason for this is simple. When you fast and have lesser hours of feeding, your body will be running on less energy, making you feel tired. Additionally, since fasting can boost stress levels, it is also likely to disrupt your sleep patterns. To counter this, avoid doing too many activities or even try meditating. If you follow a regular fitness routine, you need to schedule your workouts to the times when you get to eat. This makes it possible to have a pre and post work out meal. Besides, working out when fasting may result in low blood sugar levels with symptoms like confusion and dizziness in addition to putting you at risk of injuries.

## You Might Be Dehydrated

The thing about intermittent fasting is that when you stop eating during the fasting window, you might also be unable to remember about drinking up. When you forget to drink water, you will end up being dehydrated. This may be interpreted as hunger so much so that you end up giving in to the cravings.

## You Might Feel Hungry

When you set out to do intermittent fasting, you will notice that your stomach will start grumbling after the first few hours of fasting because your body is used to being fed after a few hours. However, you can take action to keep hunger in check so that you don't interfere with your intermittent fasting plan. Among the things you can do is avoid the thought or even smell of food that is likely to trigger the production of gastric acid in the stomach, making you feel hungry. You can consider finding various distractions, such as reading a book or getting involved in an activity that is mentally engaging. Taking water and beverages that do not contain calories will also fill your stomach, making you pull through the fasting window.

The other way to deal with hunger pangs is making sure that you take advantage of your eating periods by opting for a diet that is nutritionally balanced. This includes food laden with fiber to keep you feeling full for longer, as well as protein and healthy fats. Above all, start slow. You can begin intermittent fasting for a week and see how well it blends into your schedule as well as how your body responds as well as how well your fasting schedule fits into your lifestyle. Ultimately, you need to find what works for you.

## You Might Feel Irritable

The hormones that regulate your appetite are also

responsible for regulating your mood. Your nutrient consumption affects the activity levels of your neurotransmitters like serotonin and dopamine that play a role in both depression and anxiety. This means that dysregulating your appetite could turn your mood around. You will do well to stick to a diet that is not only nutritionally balanced but also satiating during your feasting window. You should also ensure you're getting enough sleep because it is also linked to your mood.

## You Might Feel Cold

When you fast, the flow of blood to your fat stores will tend to increase. Consequently, your blood sugar levels will begin to decrease so that you're more sensitive to feeling cold, especially your hands and toes. This is a common feeling; however, you need to make sure you dress properly.

## Your Might Have Constipation, Heartburn, and Bloating

The stomach produces acid that is very important to the digestion process. This means that you could experience heartburn when this acid is released, and you're not eating. As a result, you could experience some discomfort and burping. To avoid this, make sure you take adequate water while avoiding foods that are greasy and spicy.

## You Might Have Headaches

Failing to sufficiently hydrated when you're doing intermittent fasting may result in headaches. Therefore, always make sure that you're drinking up enough water as other non-caloric fluids, whether you're within your fasting or feasting window.

## You Might Have Cravings

When you go for extended periods without food, you could begin to have cravings for processed carbohydrates and sweet foods because your body needs glucose to keep you going.

## You Might Have Poor Weight Management

When you practice intermittent fasting, it's unlikely that you will be able to manage your weight properly. This is because you could have cravings for certain calories that you may end up overindulging when it's time to eat. This will eventually be counterproductive to your intermittent fasting efforts.

## Long-Term Downsides

When you fast for extended durations, your immune system may be compromised, eventually affecting your vital organs like the kidneys and liver. When you stay for long before eating, you may end up with malnourishment that can end up in untimely death when not checked.

Overall, you should expect your body to react to withdrawal or abstaining from eating. While you will get used to the short term effects such as outbursts, weakness, dizziness, and low blood pressure, make sure you don't overlook serious intermittent fasting risks.

# Chapter 9:

# What Is Keto Diet?

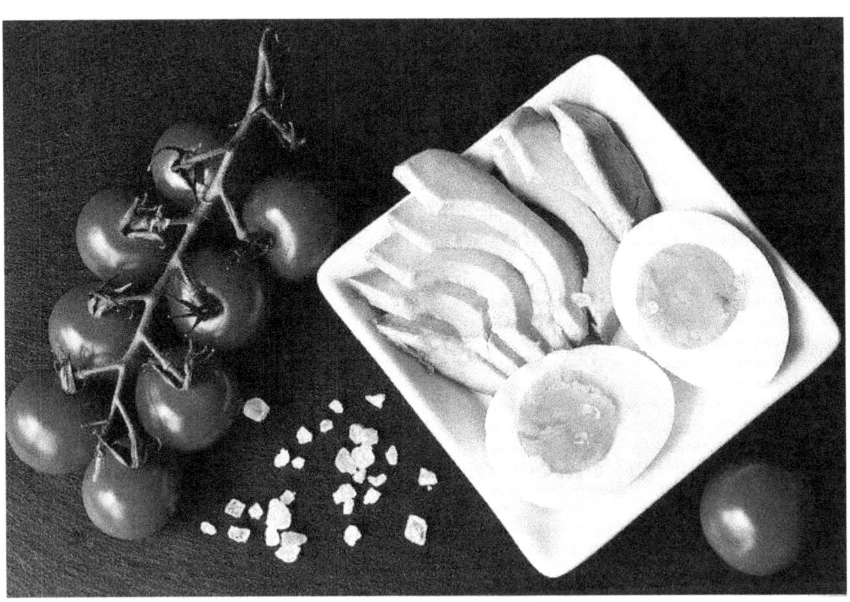

The ketogenic diet refers to a diet that emphasizes on taking low carbs and high fats ostensibly to gain many health benefits. Several studies have shown that this diet is able to help you to lose weight, thus improving your health. The ketogenic diet is based on the fact that when you withhold carbohydrates, your body will be forced to turn to an alternative source of energy by burning fuel that is stored in the form of fat, thus promoting weight loss. When you eat foods that are high in carbohydrates, your body will convert the carbs into blood sugar or glucose that is then used as energy. Since glucose is the simplest form of energy that the body uses, it is always used even before your body can turn to the stored fats for fuel.

Therefore, when you go on a ketogenic diet, the idea is to restrict the consumption of carbohydrates so that the body has no choice but to break down the stored fat to obtain energy. When this happens, the fat is usually broken down within the liver, thus producing ketones that are by-products of metabolic processes. These ketones will then be used where there is no glucose as a source of energy. This process is known as ketosis. When ketosis takes place, your body will become efficient in burning fat as a source of energy that is supplied to the brain; Ketogenic diets are capable of causing massive reductions in insulin and blood sugar levels thus bringing along numerous health benefits.

# How Does the Ketogenic Diet Work?

To understand how the ketogenic diet works, it is important to begin by understanding the fat-burning mechanism behind this diet. Generally speaking, the ketogenic diet pegged on the idea of getting your body into ketosis so as to maximize fat loss. Ketosis is a normal metabolic process that takes place whenever the body does not have enough glucose stores for energy. Whenever these stores are depleted, your body will tune to burning fat as a source of energy. It is during this process that acids referred to as ketones are produced that then build up in the body for use as energy. How then can you tell if you're in ketosis? One of the ways of determining whether you are in a state of ketosis is by looking at your urine to see if there are any ketones. You can do a quick test using ketone strips that are available at retail stores. If a ketone strip does test positive for ketones, then it means that you are in a state of ketosis.

However, most people try to link the high presence of ketones to a diabetic medical emergency that is referred to as ketoacidosis. It is important to keep in mind that the nutritional ketosis that is linked to a ketogenic diet is quite different from ketoacidosis. Why is this a major concern? A rapid increase in the ketone levels in people who have diabetes may signal a health crisis that must be attended to immediately. When the insulin hormone is not sufficient, the body is unable to use the glucose that is available for fuel. Thus, the body will turn to burn stored fat for energy through the ketosis process. This leads to the building up of ketones in the body. When these ketones accumulate in the bloodstream of a person living with diabetes, the blood becomes more acidic, hence ketoacidosis. This condition can be potentially fatal and thus should be treated immediately.

## How Can Keto Help People with Type 2 Diabetes

Diabetes is a medical condition that is characterized by high blood pressure, impaired insulin function, and changes in metabolism. The ketogenic diet has been found to help in losing excess fat that is closely correlated to type 2 diabetes, metabolic syndrome, and diabetes. A study conducted on the effects of the keto diet on diabetes showed this diet contributed to improved insulin sensitivity by up to 75%. Another study with 21 participants with type 2 diabetes followed the ketogenic diet, and 7 were able to stop using medications for diabetes. In yet another research, those who followed the keto diet lost 24.4 pounds compared to 15.2 pounds lost by those who were on a high-carb diet. Furthermore, 95.2% of these participants stopped or reduced the use of diabetes medication.

The fact that the ketogenic diet is based on cutting consumptions of carbs, it's commonly used in controlling blood sugar. In fact, this diet has become quite popular among people who have type 2 diabetes and are looking to lower their A1C. That is the average measurement of their blood sugar levels over a period of two to three months. According to research, the ketogenic diet could lead to fast weight loss as well as potentially low blood sugar for people who have the disease. However, dieticians also warn that the ketogenic diet also presents a number of risks, particularly among those people who are living with and managing diabetes. These include potential low blood sugar as well as possible drug interactions if you're on medication. In some cases, it could also result in kidney damage, especially in those people who have dysfunctional kidneys because of an elevated amount of ketones in the bloodstream. If you want to try the ketogenic diet while managing diabetes, it is important that you do so after consulting your healthcare provider, so make sure that it's safe and effective.

## Types of Ketogenic Diet

The ketogenic diet can be practiced in different variations even though only two of these have been studied extensively. The four different kinds of intermittent fasting are:

## The Standard Ketogenic Diet (SKD)

This type of ketogenic diet is targeted for weight loss, healing disease, as well as therapeutic purposes. When following this plan, you will plan all your snacks and meals around fat, such as olive oil, olives, meats, fatty fish, ghee, butter, and avocados. Overall, you must get at least 150 grams of fat per day to be able to shift your metabolism so that your body can get to burn fat as fuel. You will also need to cut on your carbs from 300 grams daily to not more than 50 grams. This essentially means you will have to stick to non-starchy veggies, leafy vegetables/greens, as well as low-carb fruits like melon and berries. You will also have to eat moderate proteins that are about 90 grams daily or portion it to 30 grams per meal.

## The Targeted Ketogenic Diet (TKD)

This type of ketogenic diet is designed for those who want increased work outperformance because it is holistic. As such, this form of the ketogenic diet is quite popular among athletes as well as individuals who are active and live on a keto lifestyle but with more carbs. This diet allocates an additional 20-30 grams of carbs immediately before and after workouts. This allows for you to be able to sustain higher intensity exercise as well as enhanced recovery. Thus, the total amount of carbs consumed per day is between 70 and 80 grams. The best food options for this diet include dairy, fruit, or grain-based foods, as well as sports nutrition products. Since any additional carbs are quickly burned off, there is no room for storage in the body as fat.

# The High-Protein Keto Diet (HPKD)

This diet is perfect if you have high-protein needs. This diet plan entails eating about 120 grams for protein daily as well as 130 grams of fat daily. Even then, carbs are still restricted to less than 10% of your daily calorie consumption. Most people find this modified keto easy to follow since it allows you to eat more protein and less fat compared to the standard ketogenic diet. However, you need to take caution with this approach because it might not result in ketosis. The reason for this that the proteins are converted to glucose for fuel, just like carbs. Following this diet will, however, result in weight loss.

# The Cyclical Ketogenic Diet (CKT)

The cyclical ketogenic diet is recommended for professional athletes and bodybuilders. It involves following the standard ketogenic diet for at least 5 or 6 days a week before following up with higher carbohydrate consumption for the next 1 to 2 days. The days when you get to consume a higher amount of carbs are referred to as refeeding days because they are meant for replenishing the depleted glucose reserves. When you follow this ketogenic diet approach, you will switch from ketosis during the refeeding days so as to tap into the benefits of temporary carb consumption. Those who want to improve their exercise performance and attain muscle growth mostly practice this type of ketogenic diet.

Although the cyclical ketogenic diet is usually compared to carb cycling, it's not the same thing. Carb cycling is different in that it involves cutting carbs on specific days of the week while increasing your intake on other days. Each week is often divided in 4 to 6 days of lower carbs and another 1 to 3 days of a higher intake. Although this method is the same, the difference is that carb cycling does not reduce the overall intake of carbohydrates drastically for the body to attain ketosis. To get the best results with the cyclical ketogenic diet, you need to eat wholesome carbohydrate-rich foods on the days when you're off. This includes dairy products, starchy veggies, fruits, whole grains, and dairy products.

# Ketogenic Diets and Weight Loss

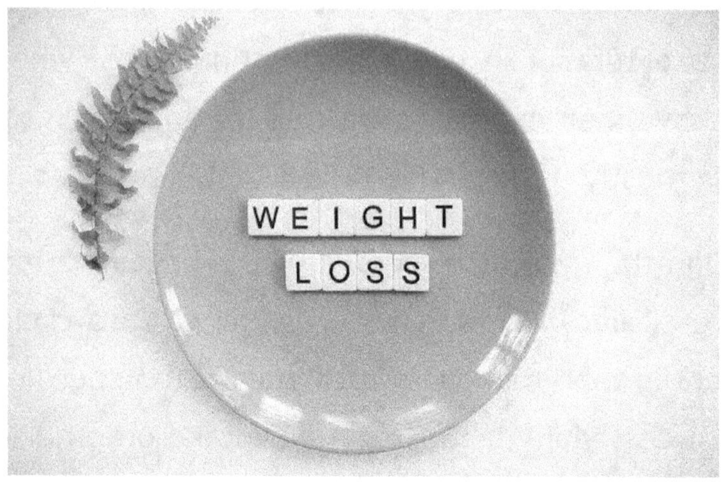



The ketogenic diet is an effective way of losing weight as well as lowering risk factors for various diseases. According to research, the ketogenic diet is quite superior and is often recommended compared to the low-fat diet. This diet is more filling so that you are able to lose weight even without having to keep track of the calories you consume. According to one study, people who followed the ketogenic diet lost 2.2 times more weight compared to those who followed a calorie-restricted low-fat diet. Moreover, the HDL and triglyceride levels of those who followed the keto diet also improved. In another study, people who followed the ketogenic diet lost 3 times more weight compared to those on a diet that was recommended by Diabetes. Some of the reasons that make the ketogenic diet superior include the increase in protein intake that has several benefits. The increase in ketones, improved insulin sensitivity, and low blood sugar levels also play an important role.

## Getting Started on the Ketogenic Diet

There are a number of things you need to know before you get started with the ketogenic diet. First, following the diet requires a drastic restriction of carbohydrates from your diet as you carefully monitor your food choices to ensure that you're meeting your nutritional needs. You will do well to work closely with a registered dietician as they will help you to make sure that you implement this plan well while minimizing the risk for potential complications or side effects. It's also important to keep in mind the goal of making this dietary change is promoting a healthy lifestyle; therefore, make sure you select a meal plan that you can stick to in the long term. If you will be unable to follow the plan in the long term, then this diet is probably not meant for you.

# Chapter 10: Intermittent Fasting and Ketogenic Diet

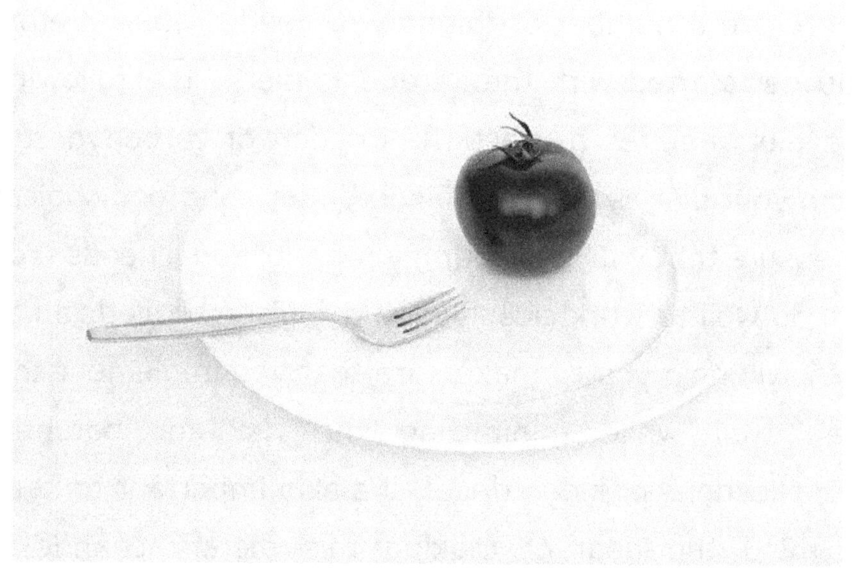

Intermittent fasting and the ketogenic have both grown in popularity in health enthusiasts, as well as people who want to lose weight over the years. There are just as many people who are attracted to intermittent fasting as there are in ketogenic diets, obviously because of the promising health benefits the two offer. Over time, those who want to tap into both intermittent fasting and keto have come up with a combination of the two. Thus, it's possible to tap into the benefits of both because they go hand in hand. Intermittent fasting and the ketogenic diet complement each other very well.

## The Difference Between Intermittent Fasting and the Ketogenic Diet

Before getting to know how intermittent fasting and ketogenic diet work together, it's important first to understand the key differences between the two. While intermittent fasting is more about when you should eat your food, the ketogenic diet limits the consumption of carbs while emphasizing the consumption of high-fat foods and moderate proteins. When you take part in intermittent fasting, you will prolong the periods you will go without food to between 16 and 24 hours, depending on the intermittent fasting method you will select. However, you can take plenty of water as well as plain coffee and tea during this time.

During intermittent fasting, you will have a feeding

window and a fasting window. You can begin by fasting for fewer hours and expanding your fasting window gradually. Focusing on the keto-friendly foods during your feeding window will help in prolonging helpful metabolic pathways that are invoked during fasting. Ultimately, both methods of dieting work towards the goal of getting the body to use fat stores for their energy and getting the body in the state of ketosis. Both intermittent fasting and keto diet deplete body glucose so that your body gets into ketosis faster than it would when you depend on fasting alone.

## Why Should You Combine Intermittent Fasting and Keto?

Doing intermittent fasting and keto can help with weight loss in the short term. However, since both diets are restrictive, they are certainly not for everyone. So does combining them post better results than following eat plan separately?

Some experts hold the view that it is better to combine intermittent fasting and keto. While the keto diet will increase the levels of ketones in your body, intermittent fasting also sees an increase in ketones. The brain will not overly rely on glucose for energy when it is in a state of nutritional ketosis. Thus, the transition into ketosis will become seamless when you're on a low-carb ketogenic diet. Adding intermittent fasting will definitely take things a notch higher. This may include overcoming the weight loss plateau because you may eat fewer calories when doing intermittent fasting. Intermittent fasting keto may also be a form of a natural progression from the keto diet, especially if you feel satiated eating so much fat and are not bothered reducing the eating window.

## Who Can Follow Intermittent Fasting Keto?

Intermittent fasting keto is ideal for anyone who has been following the keto diet for more than two weeks and have the approval of your health care professional. However, intermittent fasting keto will most certainly be a no go zone for you if you have a history of an eating disorder, have chronic kidney diseases, or are undergoing active treatment for cancer. Pregnant and nursing mothers may also not practice intermittent fasting. In fact, you may not practice either of these diets at all. Additionally, if you are following a keto diet and are happy with the results or you feel good about the way you're progressing, then you might not need intermittent fasting.

## Benefits of Fasting on the Ketogenic Diet

There's a significant overlap between intermittent fasting and the ketogenic diet. Here are some of the health benefits of intermittent fasting and why you should consider fasting when on a low-carb diet.

## Intermittent Fasting Enables Your Body to Enter Ketosis Faster

Intermittent fasting works this way; when your body is in the fasted state, it will begin to burn the fat stores in order to access energy. This is similar to the process that takes place before your body enters into ketosis. When the glucose in your body is depleted, your body begins to burn the fat stores or ketone to obtain energy. However, when given a choice, your body will tap energy from glucose as its primary source at any given time. This means that by restricting your intake of carbohydrates significantly, your body will switch to burning ketones through a metabolic process referred to as ketosis. Sometimes, following a low-carb and high-fat diet is not usually enough; therefore, intermittent fasting can help to hasten the process of entering into ketosis. Fasting also helps to deplete your glycogen stores faster so that you enter the ketogenic state.

## Intermittent Fasting on Keto Will Help You to Lose Weight Faster

One of the reasons why most people opt to complement intermittent fasting with the ketogenic diet is because it helps to lose weight much faster. Intermittent fasting alone has gained prominence for the mere reason that it's an excellent way to lose fat and weight. Combining intermittent fasting and the ketogenic diet will help you to break free from the weight loss plateaus in a number of ways. Having a shorter eating window will help in eliminating unnecessary snacking, particularly late into the night. Moreover, your body is able to comfortably accommodate a certain amount of calories at any given time; therefore, by limiting your feeding window, you also limit your daily intake of calories. Finally, when you are on a high-fat keto diet, the process of ketosis will reduce your appetite while increasing your satiety levels. This makes it much easier to practice intermittent fasting compared to when you're on a diet full of carbs that are likely to increase your need for snacking and cravings.

## Intermittent Fasting on Keto Will Help You to Avoid Keto Flu

If you have never been on the ketogenic diet before, intermittent fasting will come in handy to help you in avoiding or managing some of the uncomfortable side effects of keto that include the keto flu. These side effects often occur when your body is transitioning to the fat-burning state. How then does intermittent fasting help in negating the keto flu? Well, since the keto flu will most certainly occur when you get into ketosis and tends to go away as soon as your metabolic switch is activated, you're less likely to experience the negative effects of ketosis if you can get into ketosis faster. The fact that a short fast is able to help you to get into ketosis, it can also help to reduce the likelihood of suffering from the keto flu.

# Intermittent Fasting on Keto Helps the Body to Heal Itself

Intermittent fasting activates a process that is referred to as autophagy, which is a phenomenon that helps in healing the body. This process essentially promotes a cleansing process that eliminates and recycles all the dead and broken proteins, among other unwanted cells. The process of autophagy may be triggered during the windows of starvation when carbohydrates are restricted and could help the body to heal itself of chronic diseases like cancer.

# Intermittent Fasting on Keto Helps in Stabilizing Your Blood Sugar

One of the benefits of intermittent fasting is that it helps in striking a balance in your insulin levels. When you get rid of sugar and carbs from your diet, you are effectively eliminating the possibility of blood sugar spikes that will often come with eating these foods. If you're looking to control your blood sugar levels, fasting on keto will go a long way in helping find a balance. Fasting also helps to improve insulin sensitivity as well as prevent insulin resistance that can reduce your chances of developing type 2 diabetes or heart disease.

# Tips to Help You Manage Intermittent Fasting Keto

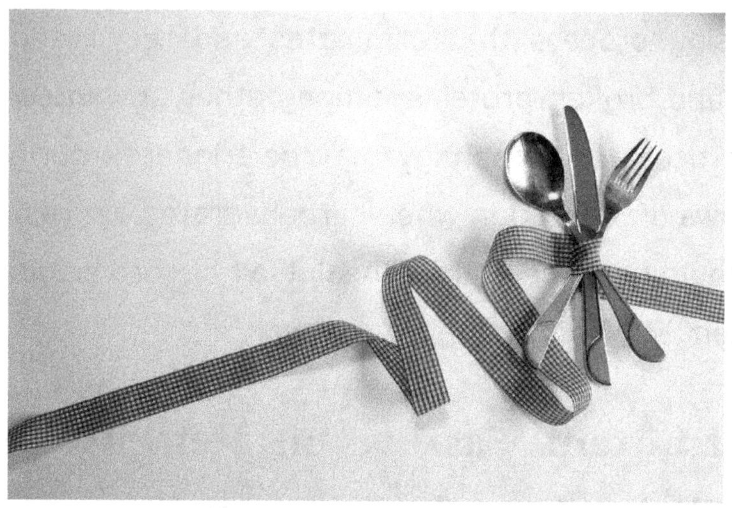

The truth is that it can be quite tricky at the beginning when you start experimenting on combining intermittent fasting and keto. Here are some tips to help you if you want to start on intermittent fasting keto and succeed:

## Measure Your Ketone Levels

Although fasting will help you to stay in ketosis, you still need to make sure that you are not eating too many carbs or doing anything that might get you out of ketosis. When you track your ketone levels, you will be able to ensure that you are actually in ketosis.

## Make Sure You're Eating Enough

When you go for extended durations without food, you may naturally eat fewer calories throughout the day. This could easily result in deficiencies in vitamins or even the development of metabolic issues; therefore, make sure your calorie intake is at a level that is considered healthy. Severe restriction of calories could lead to the loss of muscle mass, along with depleted levels of energy and other side effects that are unhealthy. Even then, you shouldn't take advantage of short fasts to eat sugary or carbohydrate-laden foods or go through phases of overeating. Rather your focus should be on nutrient-dense foods. You will do well to consider following a keto meal plan so that you eat plenty of healthy foods such as coconut oil, avocado, and MCT oil, plenty of leafy green vegetables and high-quality proteins from both plant and animal-based sources.

# Begin with a Moderate Approach

If you are new to intermittent fasting, you will do well to consider beginning with by skipping a meal and slowly extending your fasting window. During this time, you will be observing how your body responds and if there are any negative side effects before you can finally transition to a full fast.

# How to Start on Intermittent Fasting Keto

It's advisable that you don't begin intermittent fasting and keto at the same time. The reason for this is that you will shock your system because it will be switching from glucose as the primary source of fuel to ketone. Moreover, implementing intermittent fasting in itself is a significant change. For this reason, it is common for most people to begin with keto and only consider combining it with intermittent fasting after a couple of weeks or even months.

The most important thing you need to consider is choosing the right timing. A 12- to 16-hour fast is recommended in most cases because, for most people, it's almost natural not to eat for 12 hours because most hours are covered at night when you're sleeping. Moreover, this will not require any meal skipping. To start off, you need to consider delaying your breakfast by an hour and extend gradually. This will help in getting your body accustomed to going for longer durations without eating.

Once you've settled into your new pattern of eating, you can reintroduce breakfast earlier in the day and extend your fasting time because eating breakfast will not only lead to better cognition but also helps to improve insulin sensitivity and metabolism. How long it will while you follow intermittent fasting keto should not be more than six months after which you transition back to a standard low-carb diet.

In general, intermittent fasting is a practice that involves going without food for a designated period. Since intermittent fasting depletes your glycogen stores, it's great for complementing a keto diet. However, you must begin with a moderate approach because both keto and intermittent fasting can be too harsh on your body. Intermittent fasts offer benefits that are similar to keto, such as weight and fat loss, balanced sugar levels, and accelerating the process of ketosis. You need to make sure you give your body adequate time to adjust while eating the foods that are outlined in the keto plan. Intermittent fasting and keto diet both have risks associated with them; therefore, you need to make sure that you're doing it right to minimize the risks key among them being nutritional deficiencies.

# Chapter 11:

# Benefits of the Ketogenic Diet and Getting into the State of Ketosis

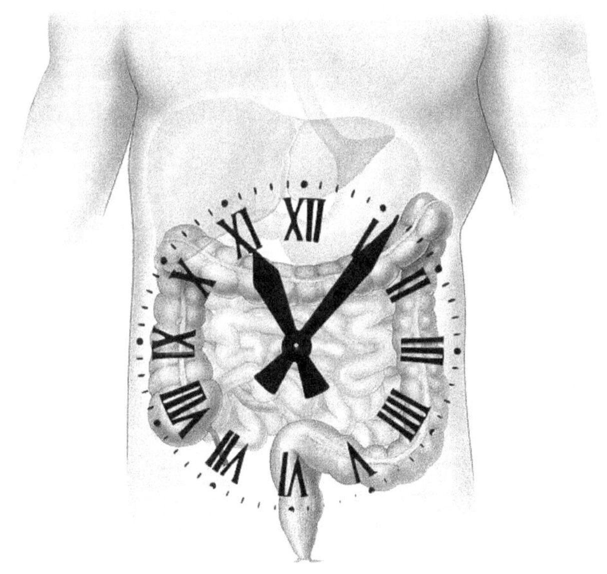

What makes the ketogenic diet a good consideration for you? Low-carb diets have attracted a fair share of controversy over the years. However, numerous scientific studies have been done to prove the worth of these diets and found them to be both beneficial and healthy.

## Benefits of the Ketogenic Diet

Here are some of the benefits of following the ketogenic diet:

## Low-Carb Diets Will Reduce Your Appetite

One of the worst side effects of dieting is hunger. In fact, this is one of the reasons why most people tend to give up on diets because they end up being miserable. On the contrary, low-carb eating will result in an automatic reduction in your appetite. Studies have shown that when people reduce their intake of carbs and instead eat more protein and fat, they end up eating fewer calories altogether.

## Low-Carb Diets Will Enhance More Weight Loss Initially

Reducing your intake carbs is one of the easiest yet most

effective ways of losing weight. Studies have demonstrated that people who followed a low-carb and high-fat diet tend to shed off more weight a lot faster than those who follow other low-fat diets that mostly focus on restricting calorie consumption. This is linked to the fact that low-carb diets act to eliminate excess water from the body and lower your level of insulin resulting in rapid loss of weight within the first or second week. In studies that have compared low-fat and low-carb diets, those who restrict carbs will, in some instances, lose 2-3 times as much weight even without having to feel hungry. A study carried out in adults who were obese found that a low-carb diet is effective up to about six months compared to the conventional weight loss diet, after which the difference is inconsequential.

## Low-Carb Diets Lead to a Drastic Decline in Triglycerides

Triglycerides refer to the fat molecules that are found in the bloodstream. When these triglycerides are high in the blood, they are a strong risk factor for heart disease. One of the factors that could lead to an increase in the levels of triglyceride in the blood in people who lead a sedentary lifestyle is the consumption of carbohydrates. When people reduce the intake of carbs, they tend to experience a dramatic reduction in the level of triglycerides in their blood. Consequently, low-fat diets also have the potential of increasing triglyceride levels.

## Ketogenic Diets Promote the Loss of Abdominal Fat

All the fat in your body is not the same. The place where fat is stored will not only determine your risk of disease but health as well. There are two main types of fat—namely, visceral fat that accumulates within the abdominal cavity and subcutaneous fat that is found under the skin. Visceral fat often lodges around organs, with the excess being associated with insulin resistance and inflammation. In addition, it may also result in metabolic dysfunction. Low-carb diets have been found to be quite effective in reducing the amount of harmful visceral fat, as a great proportion of fat and weight loss for those on low-carb diets seems to come from the abdominal cavity. Eventually, this also results in a reduced risk of type 2 diabetes and heart disease.

# Keto Supports Reduced Blood Sugar and Insulin Levels

Low-carb diets are usually helpful for people who have insulin resistance and diabetes that affect millions of people across the world. Studies have shown that cutting carbs will lower both the insulin and blood sugar levels significantly. Some of the people who have diabetes and have started on a low-carb diet may need to reduce their dosage of insulin by up to 50% almost immediately. In a study conducted in people with type 2 diabetes, 95% had reduced or eliminated medications lowering glucose within six months. Even then, make a point of talking to your doctor if you take blood sure mediation before you can begin on the keto diet.

# Keto Diet Will Increase Your Levels of Good HDL Cholesterol

The good cholesterol is referred to as High-Density Lipoprotein (HDL). When your levels of HDL are higher compared to the levels of the bad cholesterol LDL, you have a lower risk of suffering from heart disease. Eating a low-carb diet with a lot of fat will help to increase your good HDL levels. It's not surprising that the HDL levels will dramatically increase when you follow a healthy low-carb diet and only increase when moderately or even decline when you are on low-carb diets.

## A Ketogenic Diet Is Effective Against Metabolic Syndrome

Metabolic syndrome refers to the condition that is associated with your risk of heart disease and diabetes. It's a collection of various symptoms, among them low levels of good HDL cholesterol, high triglycerides, elevated fasting blood sugar levels, abdominal obesity, and elevated blood pressure. A low-carb diet will help in treating all these symptoms resulting in the elimination of the metabolic syndrome altogether.

## A Ketogenic Diet May Lower Blood Pressure

Hypertension or elevated blood pressure is another significant risk factor for various diseases that include stroke, kidney failure, and heart disease. Low-carb diets are effective in lowering blood pressure that should effectively reduce the risk of these diseases, thus increasing your lifespan.

## A Ketogenic Diet Will Improve the Levels of Your Bad LDL Cholesterol, Thus Boosting Your Heart Health

People who have a high level of bad cholesterol have a higher risk of heart attacks. Generally, the size of the particles is significant because the smaller particles translate to a higher risk, while bigger particles translate to a lower risk. Lower carb diets will increase the size of the bad LDL cholesterol particles, thus reducing the overall number of LDL particles within your bloodstream. This will boost your heart health.

## It's Therapeutic for Several Brain Disorders

Your brains require glucose, and its only certain parts of that are able to burn the kind of sugar. This is why the liver has to produce glucose from protein if you don't consume any carbs. Interestingly another part of your brain is capable of burning ketones that form when you're starved, and your carb intake is low. This is how the ketogenic diet works, a mechanism that has been used for decades in the treatment of epilepsy in children who don't show improvement with drug treatment. In most cases, this diet is able to cure children of epilepsy as one study found out that children who were put on the ketogenic diet had a 50% reduction in the frequency of seizures, with 16% becoming seizure-free.

## A Ketogenic Diet Can Help to Reduce the Risk of Cancer

Studies have shown that the ketogenic diet is a great way of preventing or even treating certain kinds of cancers. In one study, findings show that the ketogenic diet may be suitable as a complementary form of treatment to chemotherapy as well as radiation in people who have cancer. This is linked to the fact that going on a ketogenic diet will result in oxidative stress in the cancer cells than in the ordinary cells. Other theories suggest that since the ketogenic diet will reduce your blood sugar levels, it can help in reducing insulin complications that are associated with certain cancers.

# A Ketogenic Diet Helps to Reduce Acne

There are various causes of acne, and one may be related to blood sugar or diet. Eating a diet that is high in refined and highly processed carbohydrates may alter gut bacteria and result in more dramatic fluctuations in your blood sugar. These can have an impact on your skin health. Thus, when you decrease your intake of carbs, you could as well end up with a reduction in acne.

# Ketogenic Diet Improves Health in Women Who Suffer from Polycystic Ovarian Syndrome (PCOS)

The polycystic ovarian syndrome (PCOS) refers to an endocrine disorder that causes the ovaries to enlarge with cysts. Women who suffer from this disorder are likely to experience negative effects from consuming a high-carbohydrate diet. Although there are few clinical studies on the ketogenic diet and PCOS, one study involving 5 women over 24 weeks found that the ketogenic diet aided hormone balance, increased weight loss, improved the amount of fasting insulin, and improved the ratio of the follicle-stimulating hormone and the luteinizing hormone.

## How to Get in Ketosis Fast

Achieving ketosis not always easy. Although most people who desire to attain ketosis will adhere to the ketogenic diet, there are different other ways through which you can get into ketosis fast. Here are some tips to help you get into ketosis:

## Elevating Your Physical Activity Level

If you use more energy during the day, you will need to eat more food in order to be energetic. Exercise will help you to deplete your glycogen stores in their bodies. In most instances, the glycogen stores become replenished whenever you eat carbohydrates. This means that when you're on a low-carb diet, these stores will not be replenished. It may take time before the body learns how to use fat stores instead of glycogen; hence, you may experience fatigue during the period when the body will be going through an adjustment.

# Reducing Your Carbs Intake Significantly

Ketosis will take place when the absence of carbohydrates forces the body to use fat as the primary source of energy in the place of glucose. Whether you're looking to attain ketosis for weight loss or you simply want to reduce the risk of heart disease or even control and maintain blood sugar levels, you should aim at reducing your consumption of carbohydrates to a maximum of 20 grams daily. Even then, this number is not cast in stone; thus, you may need to do a little more carbs yet still manage to enter ketosis, while others may need less.

# Practicing Short Fasts

Fasting or going for a couple of hours without consuming any calories may actually lead to ketosis. In controlled cases, a doctor could recommend longer fasting durations of between 24 and 48 hours. It is important to first talk to your doctor before making the decision to fast for longer durations. Fat fasting is a kind of fasting that involves reducing your calorie intake significantly and only eating a diet that consists of fat for not more than 2 or 3 days. According to research, this will have a significant effect on your weight loss efforts. The challenge is that it's difficult to sustain fat fasting making it less favorable for most people.

## Testing Ketone Levels

One of the ways of getting to attain ketosis is by monitoring the levels of ketones in your body. You can do this by performing a number of tests that include breath, urine, and blood test. Using one or more of these tests will help you to keep track of your progress, thus allowing you to make educated adjustments in your diet.

## Increasing Your Intake of Healthy Fat

As your intake of carbs decreases, you need to increase your intake of fats. Some of the fats you can consider increasing include olive oil, coconut oil, flaxseed, avocadoes, and avocado oil, among others. Even then, if your overall goal is to lose weight, then you must also keep the overall consumption in mind.

# Maintain High Protein Consumption

It is important that you eat sufficient amounts of protein all through the day when you want to achieve ketosis. Protein provides two essential health benefits when you want to lose weight. That is, it helps in maintaining your muscle mass or provide amino acids to the liver to ensure proper functioning. You may experience loss of muscle mass if your intake of protein is not sufficient.

# Consuming More Coconut Oil

Increasing your intake of coconut oil could help you to attain the state of ketosis. A study conducted with the focus on Alzheimer's diseases showed that adding coconut oil in your diet can help to increase the ketone levels. Coconut oil is rich in fats known as medium-chain triglycerides (MCTs). The body is able to absorb MCTs easily and quickly. It then sends these fats to your liver, where they are turned into energy or ketones.

Ketosis is a natural state that the body needs to be in occasionally. When ketosis occurs, the body will but all the fat reserves to be used as energy. Maintaining ketosis over a short period comes with minimal risk even though people who have type 1 diabetes need to avoid ketosis, as it will only increase the risk of complications.

# Chapter 12:

# Foods You Can Eat on Keto Diet

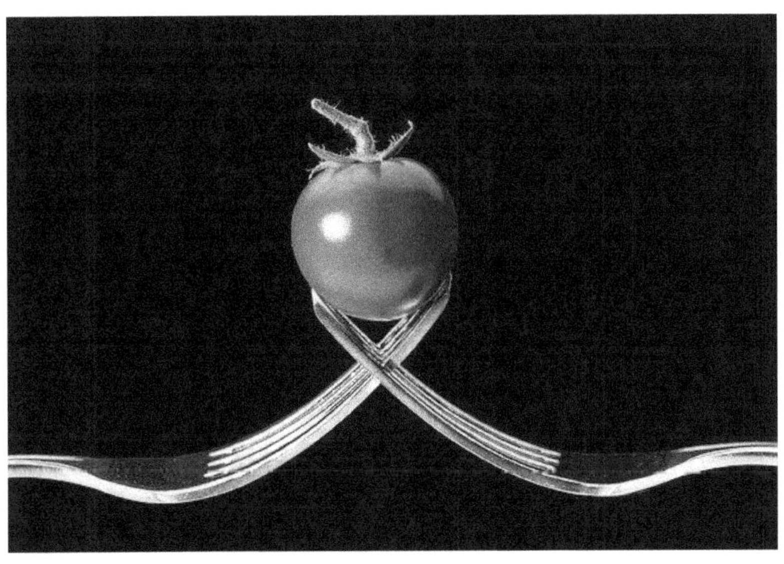

By now, you know that the ketogenic diet is high-fat and very low-carbohydrate with moderate protein. Carbohydrates are a preferred source of energy for the body, yet when you're on a strict keto diet, less than 5 % of the food you eat will account for carbohydrates. Although it may seem straight forward on what you need to eat while following this diet, the choice of foods can be confusing. Here's a guide to the foods you eat, as well as the foods you need to avoid when you're on the keto diet.

# Foods to Eat on the Ketogenic Diet

## Low-Carb Vegetables

There are various options of non-starchy vegetables that are low in carbs and calories that you can include in your keto diet. These vegetables are also great sources of various nutrients that include minerals and vitamin c. In addition, they also have antioxidants that help in protecting you against several cell-damaging free radicals. In the best-case scenario, you need to opt for non-starchy vegetables that contain less than 8g of net carbs for each cup. This means the total carbs minus fiber. Some of the low-carb vegetable choices that fit the bill include spinach, zucchini, bell peppers, green beans, cauliflower, and broccoli.

## Seafood and Fish

Fish is a rich source of selenium, potassium, and B

vitamins. This is in addition to being carb-free and protein-rich. Sardines, mackerel, salmon, albacore tuna as well as other fatty fish have high levels of omega 3 fats. These have been found to lower blood sugar levels while increasing insulin sensitivity. Frequent consumption of fish has been associated with improved mental health and a decrease in the risk of chronic diseases. You should aim to eat at least 3-ounce servings of fatty fish twice a week.

## Cheese

Cheese is high in fats, yet it has no carbs. This makes it an excellent choice for the ketogenic diet. Cheese is also rich in calcium and protein with a single slice of cheese, delivering 30 percent of your daily recommended amount of saturated fats. If you have concerns about heart disease, you'll do well taking your cheese in small portions.

## Avocados

Avocado is an excellent source of heart-friendly fats that are monosaturated. This fruit also contains potassium, a mineral that most Americans lack. Eating half of a medium avocado will give you about 9 grams of total carbohydrates and 7 grams of fiber. Plant fats like avocado do help to improve your triglyceride and cholesterol levels.

## Plain Greek Yogurt and Cottage Cheese

Cottage cheese and yogurt are calcium and protein-rich. Taking 5 ounces of plain Greek yogurt will provide you about 12 grams of proteins and 5 grams of carbohydrates. An equivalent amount of cottage cheese contains 18 grams of proteins and 5 grams of carbohydrates. Studies have found that both protein and calcium have the ability to promote fullness and reduce appetite. Hence, taking cottage cheese and higher-fat yogurts while on the keto diet will help you to stay full for longer.

## Poultry and Meat

Meat is a great source of lean proteins and a staple on the ketogenic diet. Poultry and fresh means do not contain any carbohydrates and are excellent sources of B vitamins and various minerals that include zinc, selenium, and potassium. Although you can take processed meats like sausage and bacon while on the keto diet, they are not the best for your heart and are likely to increase the risk of certain types of cancer when consumed in large quantities—thus, always choose beef, chicken, and fish while limiting processed meats.

## Nuts, Seeds, and Healthy Oils

Seeds and nuts are packed with healthy monosaturated and polyunsaturated fats, protein, and fiber. They are also low in net carbs. Coconut oil and olive oil are the two oils that are recommended when you're on the keto diet. Coconut oil is high in saturated fat nut has medium-chain triglycerides (MCTs) that promote ketone production. MCTs have the ability to increase metabolic rate and promoting weight loss as well as belly fat too. On the other hand, olive oil has a high amount of oleic acid, which is associated with a reduced risk of heart disease. It's important that you measure the portion sizes of any of these healthy fats when consuming them.

# Eggs

Eggs have a high proportion of minerals, antioxidants, and B vitamins. Two eggs have no carbohydrates but have 12 grams of protein. Eggs have shown to trigger hormones that are known to increase fullness while keeping blood sugar levels stable. They also contain antioxidants like zeaxanthin and lutein that help in protecting eye health.

# Unsweetened Tea and Coffee

Plain tea and coffee contain no carbohydrates, protein, or fat—making them a good pick when doing your keto diet. According to studies, coffee has been found to lower the risk of cardiovascular diseases as well as type 2 diabetes. On the other hand, tea contains antioxidants and less caffeine compared to coffee. Thus, drinking tea could actually reduce the risk of suffering from a stroke or heart attack while helping you to lose weight and boost your immune system.

# Berries

Berries are rich in antioxidants that are able to reduce

inflammation and protect you against disease. They are also low in carbs and high in fiber.

## Cocoa Powder and Dark Chocolate

If you have to take this, make sure you check the label because the number of carbs will depend on the type, as well as how much you will consume. Cocoa is referred to as a superfruit since it's rich in antioxidants. Dark chocolate contains flavonols, which have the ability to reduce the risk of heart disease by lowering blood pressure and keeping arteries.

## Butter and Cream

These are good fats to include in your ketogenic diet because they both contain trace amounts of carbs for each serving. Butter and cream were previously believed to contribute to heart disease because of their levels of saturates fat. Even then, a number of studies have shown that there is no link between saturated fat and heart disease. Other studies suggest moderate consumption of high-fat dairy could possibly reduce the risk of heart attack or stroke.

## Shirataki Noodles

These are a great addition to the ketogenic diet. They have less than one gram of carbs along with 5 calories per serving because they have water. In fact, these noodles are made from viscous fiber referred to as glucomannan, which can absorb at least 50 times the weight. The viscous fiber forms a gel that slows down food movement through the digestive tract. This can help in decreasing hunger and blood sugar spikes, thus making it quite beneficial for the weight loss process and management of diabetes.

# Foods to Avoid on a Keto Diet

## Foods That Contain Added Sugar

You must avoid any foods that contain sweeteners, as these are likely to raise your blood sugar effectively, causing your insulin levels to spike. When this happens, your appetite will also be stimulated, thus getting you out of ketosis.

# Cereals

You must avoid all grains, including whole grains like rye, wheat, oats, corn, millet, barley, sorghum, bulgur, amaranth, sprouted grains, and buckwheat. This also includes any products that are made from grains like bread, pasta, pizza, crackers, and cookies, as well as sugar and sweets, taking into account ice creams, agave syrup, sugary soft drinks, and sweet puddings.

# Vegetables That Grow Beneath the Ground

Most of the vegetables that grow beneath the ground are usually high at the start because they contain mostly carbs. It is better if you aim at consuming 12-15 net carbs from vegetables per day. Some of the vegetables you need to avoid include sweet potatoes, potatoes, baked potatoes, peas, yams, corn, parsnips, cassava, and artichoke.

# Processed Foods

You should avoid all processed foods that contain carrageenan, MSG, sulfites, wheat gluten, and BPAs.

# Artificial Sweeteners

Stay away from sweeteners that contain aspartame, sucralose, acesulfame, and saccharin because these are likely to cause cravings and have been linked to other health issues like migraines.

# Legumes

Most leguminous plants like peas and beans are high in protein as well as other vital nutrients. But they are also high in carbs. They include lima beans, chickpeas, baked beans, black beans, pinto beans, black eye peas, lentils, green peas, kidney beans, navy beans, cannellini beans, and great northern beans.

# Milk

Milk is not recommended on a keto diet for a number of reasons. It is difficult to digest, lacks the good bacteria, and may even contain hormones. Moreover, milk is also high in carbs; therefore, a small amount of milk could actually give you extra carbs.

# Tropical Fruits

These include papaya, mangoes, banana, and pineapple, among others. These tend to be very sugary and hence are high in carbs and will most likely get your body out of ketosis. You should also avoid fruit juices and even smoothies.

# Sweetened Yogurts

If you must take yogurt, make sure you stick to the plain one without any added sugars. Greek yogurt is preferred because it is higher in proteins but lower in carbohydrates compared to the regular yogurt.

# Gluten-Free Baked Goods

Gluten-free foods don't necessarily translate to carb-free. In fact, most of the gluten-free bread and even muffins usually have a higher proportion of carbohydrates, just like the traditional baked goods. Even worse, they lack fiber.

# Chips and Crackers

You also must avoid chips and crackers as well as other

processed grain-based snack foods.

The difference between the foods that you can take while on the keto diet and those that you can't take is mainly in the net carb content. This refers to the number of carbs that your body can fully absorb from grams of dietary fiber that you consume in a particular food. Because fiber is not absorbed or even used in the same manner as the net carbs, it's important to subtract the total amount of fiber from the total carbs in order to determine the number of carbs there are in the food that could limit the production of ketones. This means that keto-friendly food is low in the number of net carbs. Even then, there are some exceptions. For instance, not all vegetables are keto-friendly. More specifically, you cannot compare leafy vegetables to sweet potatoes. This is because one will definitely have a high amount of net carbs. Thus, the difference between foods that are keto-friendly and those that are not going down to the different amounts of net carbs that each contains.

# Chapter 13:

# Risks and Complications of the Keto Lifestyle

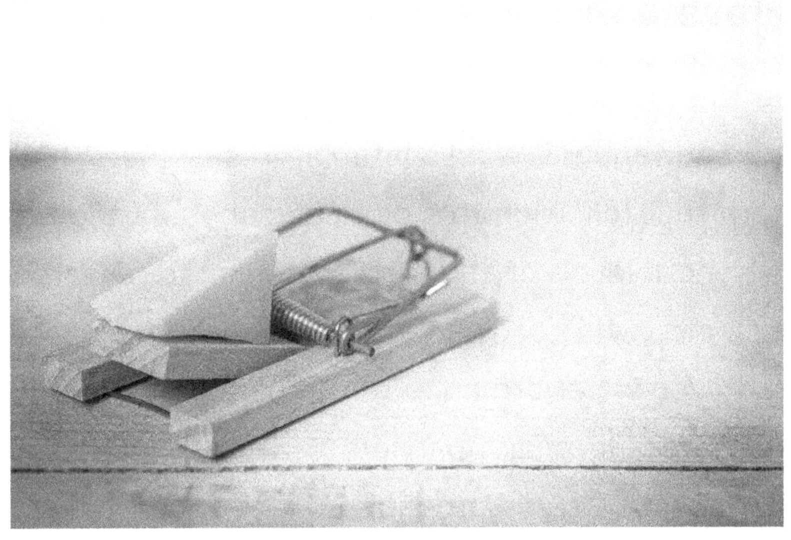

The benefits of following the ketogenic diet are quite impressive. However, there are a few risks involved. It's normal for people who start on this diet to experience various symptoms that can pass for flu, such as headaches and fatigue. So common is this side effect that it's referred to as keto flu. Yet, this diet has no signs of slowing, as it's still popular even among celebrities. It could be because this diet does not only promise quick results while letting you enjoy foods such as cheese and burgers. However, it's important to realize that this diet has its own risks that include the following:

## Keto Diet Could Affect Your Athletic Performance

While the number of athletes who have jumped on the keto bandwagon is undisputable, researchers have a concern that following this diet can sabotage the fitness and strength levels of athletes. According to researchers, participants who followed the keto diet for four days posted a poor performance on running tasks and high-intensity cycling in comparison to those who were on a high-carb diet. This is probably because, during ketosis, the body is mostly in an acidic state that is capable of limiting its ability to perform at peak levels. While keto can help athletes to lose weight that is crucial for improving speed and endurance, however, these benefits may be canceled out by a decline in the performance.

# A Ketogenic Diet May Lead to Deficiencies in Minerals and Vitamins

When you limit carbs to at least 50 grams or less per day, it means you're doing away with all unhealthy foods like refined sugar and bread. This also means that you're putting on your consumption of vegetables and fruits that are a source of carbohydrates. This raises a concern, particularly if you will be doing the keto diet for a long duration because vegetables and fruits are often very high in antioxidants as well as minerals and vitamins. This means that by eliminating them, you will end up with deficiencies in those minerals over time. In addition, it may also be difficult to get sufficient fiber as you're cutting back on the carbs because grains are a good source of fiber. As a result, you may end up with serious digestion problems from weight gain, bloating, and high blood pressure and cholesterol levels.

# You're Likely to Regain the Weight When You Relax the Rules

Let's face it. The keto diet is extremely strict, with many variations of the diet recommending that you incorporate a number of stages. The first stage is often the most intense as it involves an extremely low-carb diet, although it gives room for very few cheat days. Furthermore, it also requires that you keep track of your fat and carbohydrate performance to make sure your body enters into ketosis. Later, you can transition to the relaxed form of keto that lets you have more carbs with less monitoring. This stage is referred to as maintenance mode or keto cycling. The only problem with this approach is that you will certainly regain the weight. Although keto can be considered a great jumpstart to weight loss, the truth that it's difficult to adhere to in the long term—this can be frustrating, even though the weight you will gain back is important. Although you may have mostly lost some muscle mass initially, you will probably regain more fat and less lean muscle that not only looks and feels different on the body but will also burn calories at a slower pace. This may have an impact on your metabolism, making it difficult to lose weight in the future.

# Taking Too Much Fat Could Increase the Risk of Chronic Diseases

There is a concern about the long term effect of the keto lifestyle can affect the arteries and heart. According to a study by the American College of Cardiology, people who follow low-carb diets have a high chance of developing atrial fibrillation (AF) in comparison to those who consume carbohydrates moderately. This is the most common form of heart rhythm disorder that also raises the risk of heart failure and stroke. Another research also found that people following the low-carb and high-fat diet have a high risk of dying from cancer as well as all other causes. Even then, it's important to keep in mind that most of this research is observational such that it has only found associations with certain health outcomes and not the cause and effect relationships. More long-term research needs to be done to know just what the impact of the ketogenic diet is to the body over an extended period.

# You May Suffer Fatigue and Other Symptoms Due to Keto Flu

Keto flu is one of the most common side effects of starting on the keto diet. This is generally a combination of unpleasant symptoms that are fatigue-inducing symptoms that you may feel as the body adjusts to the reduced levels of carbohydrates. When you have keto flu, the glucose in your body begins running, forcing the body to adapt by producing and using ketones as a source of energy. Some of the common symptoms of keto flu include dizziness, fatigue, sleep problems, cramps, and palpitations. Even then, these tend to reduce and even clear as the body adjusts accordingly, usually within two weeks.

## Keto May Cause Damage to Blood Vessels

Enjoying a cheat day in the short term while following the ketogenic diet can have long term consequences. A recent study found that indulging in high sugar treats such as a bottle of soda when following a high-fat, low-carb eating place can damage your blood vessels. People who follow the keto diet for weight loss or even management of type 2 diabetes and are posting positive results could end up undoing the gains by blasting them with glucose.

## You May Experience Constipation

When you have a diet that eliminates fruits and most grains while emphasizing on fats, you may end up with gastrointestinal related side effects like constipation. This is inevitable, especially where the keto diet is not done properly.

## You May Get Diarrhea

You could find yourself running to the bathroom more often when following the ketogenic diet. This may be attributed to a number of reasons like the gallbladder being overwhelmed or lack of fiber in your diet that is common when you cut on carbs. Diarrhea may also be a result of being intolerant to dairy or sometimes the use of artificial sweeteners.

# You May Experience Unhealthy Low Blood Sugar

If you have diabetes, you must discuss any dietary changes with your healthcare provider before you jump into intermittent fasting. This is because carbs are usually broken down into glucose in the blood; hence, cutting your intake of carbohydrates could result in low levels of blood sugar. This kind of change requires proper adjustments to your insulin as well as medication so as to prevent unwanted side effects like low blood sugar, among others.

Well, while so many people can attest to the benefits of the ketogenic diet, it's important to take into account the effects and health risks that this diet possesses because if the risks outweigh the potential benefits, then you might as well consider abandoning this diet completely.

# Chapter 14: Common Intermittent Fasting Myths and Mistakes

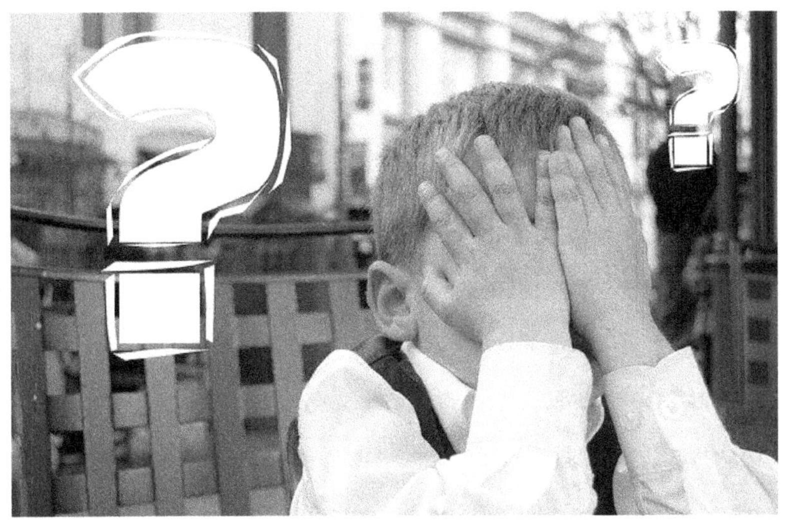

Intermittent fasting has attracted a huge following for a good reason. However, there are equally numerous myths and misconceptions surrounding this pattern of eating that only provide wrong information that can be misleading, especially for those people who want to try intermittent fasting for the first time.

## Intermittent Fasting Myths

Here are some of the common intermittent fasting myths:

# Intermittent Fasting Is Only Applicable to a Select Population

Intermittent fasting is one of the diets that can be practiced by the majority of people because it is modeled around your lifestyle. It can be tiring when you have to eat around the clock. Thus, following the intermittent fasting pattern of eating comes as a big relief because you don't have to think about what you will eat after about two to three hours. If anything, most people have schedules that favor intermittent fasting because you will not have all the time to prepare meals and sit down to eat them. Besides, it makes more sense to have three large or moderate meals than have six meals in a day.

# Intermittent Fasting Promotes Loss of Muscle

There's a widely held belief that the body needs to have a constant supply of amino acids in order to be able to repair, maintain, and even build the muscle tissue. Thus, by following the intermittent fasting diet, there will be a breakdown of your muscle tissues to obtain energy. This is not true because fasting doesn't set off your body into a catabolic mode. What those who hold this belief don't pay attention to overlook is that you can have a huge bolus of proteins that digest slowly from the last meal you had that keep on releasing amino acids enough to last the entire time of fasting.

## Intermittent Fasting Results in Binge Eating

Intermittent fasting has for long been associated with binge eating. However, it is not true that intermittent fasting will result in binge eating or any other eating disorder. When you're fasting, you need to be careful to ensure that you meet your daily macronutrient requirements. This may sometimes require you to eat a large meal, but it is in no way equivalent to binge eating, keeping in mind that this may come after working out. You need to pack up more nutrients to ensure that your daily calorie intake is met. It's impractical to imagine that you can survive on just a few raisins or nuts after following through an entire day of fasting.

# Intermittent Fasting Is Equivalent to Starvation

Fasting and starvation are not the same. Intermittent fasting is only about changing the times when you will be eating. On the other hand, starvation is extreme because the body enters starvation mode when all the stored body fat has been used up as energy. As a result, the muscles are cannibalized along with the other vital organs for survival. This can obviously not happen just because you have skipped a meal or two. If anything, your body has an immense capacity to withstand long periods of going without food during fasting bearing in mind that the body stores energy in the form of fat while the muscles serve as functional tissues.

## Frequently Eating Boosts Metabolism

Although you may eventually end up consuming fewer calories than you would normally eat, intermittent fasting is not about calorie restriction. If anything, you can plan your meals well enough to ensure that you're eating at maintenance if your goal is not weight loss. The belief that having fewer meal times slows down your metabolism is not true because you are simply postponing when you will eat. On the contrary, practicing short-time fasts can increase your resting metabolic rate.

## Intermittent Fasting Decreases Your Training Performance

Most people who are into training shy away from intermittent fasting because they believe that fasting will hamper their performance. However, a number of studies have been conducted on a number of athletes who trained during the time when they were fasting in the month of Ramadhan found that fasting doesn't stop anaerobic and aerobic performance. Remember, intermittent fasting doesn't prohibit you from taking non-caloric drinks or water. So you can stay well-hydrated for most of the day, whether you're fasting or not.

## When You Fast, You Will Feel Hungry Throughout the Entire Period of Fasting

You will not feel hungry throughout the fasting window, as it is largely assumed. The thought that you will feel hungry the entire time is mostly psychological.

Remember, you still need to go about your daily chores and activities as usual. You must make sure that you're drinking up enough fluids because both hunger and thirst are processed by the same part of the brain. You might feel hungry in the initial hours of your fast, but you will get used to it over time.

## You Can Eat Everything You Want During the Feeding Window

This is a big misconception for people who have unsuccessfully tried intermittent fasting. The fact that you have not eaten for a couple of hours doesn't mean that you can throw down pizzas and other calorie-packed meals when it is time to eat, especially if your goal is to lose weight. You must pay attention to healthy food choices because it takes time to shed off weight just like it took time to gain. Generally, eating more calories than you are supposed to will result in weight gain, thus jeopardizing your weight loss efforts.

# Women Cannot Follow the Intermittent Fasting Plan

It's assumed that just because the female body is sensitive to the starvation signals than the male body, then women can't fast. When your body senses starvation, it increases the production of leptin and ghrelin, the hormones that are responsible for controlling hunger. This will result in a feeling of insatiable hunger because this is a result of these hormones. Besides, this is the body's way of protecting a potential life even in women who are not pregnant. Women may also experience negative energy because of other reasons that include excessive stress, poor nutrition, and too little recovery, inflammation, or illnesses.

# You Should Not Take Anything During Intermittent Fasting

Some people assume that fasting is equivalent to abstaining from both food and water. In reality, you need to make sure you're well-hydrated and are free to take as much water and unsweetened tea and coffee. These are great because they contain no calories and cannot cause your insulin levels to spike. Keep in mind that the whole point of intermittent fasting is to make sure that you keep your insulin levels low.

## You Can Lose Weight with Intermittent Fasting No Matter What You Do

Many people practice intermittent fasting because they want to lose weight. But this is not always the case unless you do it the right way. Therefore, you can expect to indulge in burgers, candy, and pizza during your feasting window and lose weight. Intermittent fasting will have to work hand in hand with a healthy diet. Therefore, don't expect to lose weight if you are not focusing on healthy food choices.

## Skipping Breakfast Will Make You Lose Fat

It's widely believed that breakfast is the most important meal of the day. However, intermittent fasting allows you to skip breakfast and still be able to lead a healthy lifestyle. You'll be surprised how you can be able to have a great day despite having skipped breakfast.

# You Need to Eat Smaller Meals to Lose Weight

It's not true that eating small meals will boost your metabolism or speed up the burning of calories. In fact, taking small meals every so often will not help to reduce hunger or even the number of calories you will burn.

# Intermittent Fasting Mistakes to Avoid

Getting into intermittent fasting as a fast timer can be overwhelming because you don't really know how your body will handle it. You might end up making some mistakes that could hamper your intermittent fasting efforts. Here are some of the intermittent fasting mistakes you should avoid:

# Overeating When the Feeding Time Comes

It's easy to find yourself eating too much after hours of successful fasting just to make up for the hours you went without food. The reason for this is usually because of being emotionally starved so that you feel hungry more than you are in reality. To avoid this, you need to ensure that you carry on with your daily routine as usual, despite not eating. This is great as it will stop you from being preoccupied with your next meal when you're fasting. In addition, aim at preparing a healthy meal that is nutrient-dense as this is more satiating.

## A Fast Transition

If you have been eating after every 3-4 hours, you cannot transition to a 16-hour window suddenly as this will shock your system. As a result, you will end up with a feeling of general weakness, hunger, and discouragement to the point of giving up. Therefore, begin by fasting for fewer hours and gradually extend the fasting window until you're able to get to the 16-hour mark. This allows your body to adjust to the fasting schedule smoothly without affecting your lifestyle.

## Choosing a Wrong Intermittent Fasting Method

There are different intermittent fasting methods that you can choose to follow. However, you must make sure that you choose a method that fits into your lifestyle. Refrain from the temptation of going for an intense intermittent fasting method in the beginning. Most importantly, choose a plan that compliments your lifestyle. For instance, if you work at night, you need to go for an intermittent fasting method that allows you to eat at night so that you're fasting during the hours when you're less active.

## Failing to Take Sufficient Fluids

Intermittent fasting allows you to drink up as much fluid as possible so that you're well-hydrated. You can take water or plain tea and coffee. Avoid those fluids that contain calories and are likely to cause your insulin levels to spike because then your body will not be able to burn fat that promotes weight loss.

## Undereating During the Feeding Window

The ambition to lose weight is likely to result in eating little food when the time to eat comes. The truth is that eating too little will not facilitate more weight loss. If anything, it just might contribute to gaining weight.

When you eat too little food during your feeding window, your muscle mass will be cannibalized, thus slowing the metabolism process. The absence of metabolic muscle will interfere with your ability to process the remaining fat.

## Taking the Wrong Fluids

You must make sure that you stick to non-caloric fluids. You should avoid drinks containing sweeteners as most of these can cause a spike in insulin as well as trigger the release of the hunger hormones. You also must avoid fruit juices and alcohol since they too are packed with nutrients and sugar and are akin to eating.

## Inactivity

If you prefer having a pre-workout snack before going to the gym, you might be tempted not to engage in any activity during fasting leading to a sedentary lifestyle. What proponents of this idea forget is that the body has the ability to generate energy even after going for a few hours without food. Therefore, consider taking up an activity even if it means walking if you don't want to maintain your usual high-intensity plan. Most importantly, focus on eating foods that can help to build muscle.

## Eating Unhealthy Foods

The fact that intermittent fasting promises weight loss doesn't mean that you can indulge in all manner of calorie-packed foods. Don't use intermittent fasting as a scapegoat to eat unhealthy food. Instead, focus on eating food that is packed with nutrients. Paying attention to the nutritional value of the food you eat will help you reach your goal without having to struggle too much.

## Taking on So Many Things at the Same Time

When you resort to begin intermittent fasting, make sure you're not attempting to do many other things alongside it. This is not the time to begin following a new work out plan, taking on a new diet, or even making changes to other areas of your life. You need to focus on one thing in order to be able to track your progress and meet your goal, whatever it is. Trying to do so many things at the same time could just result in problems.

## Engaging in Intense Work Out During the Fasting Window

Although you need to make sure that you are not sedentary as you follow the intermittent fasting lifestyle, you should also avoid intense work out during the fasting window. Instead, schedule your work out during the feeding window when you are able to have a pre or post-workout meal. Don't engage in working out during the fasting window.

## Giving Up

Some people get on to the intermittent fasting bandwagon expecting quick results, and when this doesn't happen immediately, they quit. When you begin intermittent fasting, you must realize that it will take time before you get used to the new lifestyle. Moreover, while some people may begin to see the results immediately, not everyone will do because of the differences in physiology.

# Obsessing Over the Timings

In some instances, you may find yourself obsessing over the timings of your intermittent fasting plan so that all that is on your mind is when you will eat and when you will be fasting. This can get the best of you, disrupting so many aspects of your lifestyle. Instead, you need to carry on with your life as usual because the major thing that will be happening is a simple shift in your eating pattern.

# Transitioning into Intermittent Fasting

It's not everyone who starts intermittent fasting that makes it to the end with a happily ever after story. So many people start intermittent fasting only to give up along the way. Sometimes, this is a result of not making the right move when transitioning into this new way of life. Here are tips to help you make a smooth transition into intermittent fasting:

## Consult Your Doctor

This is the best place to start because your doctor needs to tell you whether you can follow this pattern of eating or not. Moreover, they will also help you to identify the right intermittent fasting method for your lifestyle. Talking to your doctor also helps to clear any doubt you may be having as they will answer all the questions you have.

## Begin with Short Fasts

You cannot make a switch from your normal routine of eating 6 times a day to fasting for 16 hours. You must ease yourself into intermittent fasting before you can begin fasting for extended hours. You can start off with an 8- to 12-hour fast and increase the fasting window over time to the point where you can fast for 16 hours comfortably.

## Eat Normally in the Initial Stages

It's impractical to make too many changes at the same time. Now that you have decided to begin on intermittent fasting, make sure there is nothing else that you are doing out of the ordinary. While you may want to overhaul your diet, you will do well to do this over time as you get used to the intermittent fasting routine. Only then can you make other changes as desired.

# Drink Plenty of Fluids

Hydration is as important to the success of your intermittent fasting as the hours you get to fast. Therefore, ensure you're taking as many fluids. This helps to give you a feeling of satiety, making it possible to cope through the hours of fasting. Besides, drinking up also helps in fighting hunger so that the hunger hormone will not send a hunger signal when you're just thirsty.

# Eat Foods That Are High in Fats and Carbs at Night

Although this may appear to counter your efforts to shed off excess weight, the truth is that it's not possible to eliminate carbs completely. Having carbs at night helps in increasing your blood sugar levels. This means that it will take time before this falls, as you will be adding it on to protein and fat. By the time your blood sugar levels dip, you will have fallen asleep. Having carbs also helps to increase the production of serotonin that leaves you feeling great after meals.

## Adhere to Your Fasting and Feeding Windows

When you start intermittent fasting, make sure you pay attention to your fasting and feasting window so that it doesn't keep in shifting. When you don't have a fixed time when you begin and end your fasting and feasting window, you confuse the body because all you will be doing is reprogramming your hunger cues each time you come up with different timing.

## Adjust Your Fasting and Feasting Times to Fit into Your Lifestyle

Whatever you do, you need to make sure that the intermittent fasting method you will select will work for you as opposed to you working for it. Therefore, you need to adjust the timings to fit into your lifestyle in terms of when you will be eating or fasting while still being able to work out and reap the benefits of intermittent fasting.

# Come Up with a Mantra That Will Serve as a Motivation

Intermittent fasting can be lonely, especially when you're doing it alone. Thus, you need to come up with creative ways to cheer yourself up so that you're able to attain your goal. One of the ways of doing this is by having a mantra that you live by. This will go a long way in improving your will power and summoning it into action. Words of affirmation and encouragement serve as a motivation to carry on even then the times seem to be toughest.

# Don't Stay Idle

You need to make sure that that you have something you're doing to keep you occupied during the day, especially if you are not working. This is a perfect way of distracting yourself from thinking about fasting and feasting or even obsess about how hungry you are. This may involve anything from attending meetings to running errands, among other things.

# Avoid Social Media Before Going to Bed

Today, social media platforms are a great way of sharing with our friends and family what we've been up to. As such, some of your friends may use their social media accounts to share their favorite recipes or even pictures of the delicious meals they have had, and this can tempt you to follow suit. You might end up being preoccupied with those images that you are unable to think about anything else other than obsessing over the feasting window.

# Manage Your Expectations

If you're getting into the intermittent fasting way of life just to lose weight, you need to approach it with realistic expectations. Being able to manage your expectations includes having the understanding that it took months of eating pizza, chocolate, and even ice cream before you put on excessive weight. Therefore, you should not expect to see the weight melt away within a short time. Being too ambitious can make you fail; instead, keep in mind that it will take time before you can start noticing the change.

## Have a Meal Plan

Although intermittent fasting doesn't have a stick meal plan to follow, and you can eat whatever healthy food you desire, you need to consider coming up with a meal plan. This will help you to stay grounded, especially with regard to your meal choices. It will also help you to ensure that you don't end up with any nutritional deficiencies that can come up because of not consuming sufficient amounts of certain foods.

## Know Your Caloric Needs

You need to make sure that you have a proper understanding of just how many calories you need to maintain your current weight or lose weight. This will inform your calorie intake so that you are certain of making progress towards the weight loss goal that you're seeking to achieve. One of the ways of establishing your calorie needs is by using the free calorie calculators that are available online. All you have to do is anonymously provide your age weight and height and let it calculate and return the results with a single click.

# Focus on Purpose

By the time you're getting into intermittent fasting, it's most likely that you have a purpose. This should serve as your driving force or an indicator that you can hold on to through the journey.

# Resist the Temptation to Overeat

When you're new to intermittent fasting, you may have the temptation to eat too much when the feasting window comes. You need to be careful so that you don't fall for this as it can result in serious complications like weight gain, bloating, and sickness.

# Track Your Progress

You need to keep a journal that helps you to keep track of the strides you're making with intermittent fasting. Journaling helps you to determine where you started and how much progress you have made. It also serves as motivation so that you stay on track and not give up.

# Conclusion

Thank you for making it through *Intermittent Fasting*! I hope this book has been able to guide you in your intermittent fasting keto journey.

Intermittent fasting and the ketogenic diet have so many similarities that make them a great combination for weight loss. Scientific studies have backed both diets by producing incredible findings that go a long way in validating these two methods of weight loss. However, you also must make sure that you're practicing intermittent fasting keto from the right environment in order to get the most out of it.

Intermittent fasting and keto diet will allow you to go for a couple of days without eating and still be able not to feel tired, lose muscle mass, or even get hungry. The keto way of life lets you shift your body into a primal state functioning, making it efficient at bioenergetics while you perform at peak. Similarly, intermittent fasting is an easy-to-implement pattern of eating that is capable of improving your life and health at the cellular level.

If you're still looking for a weight loss solution that produces results, then you need to think about combining intermittent fasting with the ketogenic diet. You only need to work a schedule that will allow you to the most out of this program. The fact that intermittent fasting can perfectly fit into your lifestyle is a reason for you to take the bold step and begin on this diet now.

What are you waiting for with all this information? The next step is to take action and implement intermittent fasting keto today. I guarantee you that when you begin this plan, your lifestyle will positively change with more motivation and you will enjoy your well-being.

Over to you now!